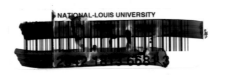

White Man's Water

White Man's Water

The Politics of Sobriety in a
Native American Community

Erica Prussing

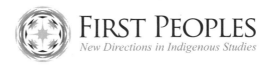

FIRST PEOPLES

New Directions in Indigenous Studies

THE UNIVERSITY OF ARIZONA PRESS
TUCSON

The University of Arizona Press
© 2011 The Arizona Board of Regents

www.uapress.arizona.edu

Library of Congress Cataloging-in-Publication Data

Prussing, Erica, 1968–
  White man's water : the politics of sobriety in a native American
community / Erica Prussing.
    p. cm.
  Includes bibliographical references and index.
  ISBN 978-0-8165-2943-8 (cloth : alk. paper)
    1. Cheyenne Indians—Alcohol use—Montana—Northern Cheyenne
Indian Reservation. 2. Cheyenne Indians—Counseling of—Mon-
tana—Northern Cheyenne Indian Reservation. 3. Cheyenne Indians—
Rehabilitation—Montana—Northern Cheyenne Indian Reservation.
4. Northern Cheyenne Indian Reservation (Mont.)—Social conditions.
I. Title.
  E99.C53P78 2011
  362.292'860897353—dc22
                                2011007999

Publication of this book was made possible, in part, with a grant from
the Andrew W. Mellon Foundation.

♻
Manufactured in the United States of America on acid-free, archival-
quality paper containing a minimum of 30% post-consumer waste and
processed chlorine free.

16   15   14   13   12   11   6   5   4   3   2   1

Figure 1, The Twelve Steps, is reprinted with permission of Alcoholics Anonymous
World Services, Inc. (AAWS). Permission to reprint the Twelve Steps does not
mean that AAWS has reviewed or approved the contents of this publication, or
that AAWS necessarily agrees with the views expressed herein. A.A. is a program
of recovery from alcoholism *only*—use of the Twelve Steps in connection with
programs and activities which are patterned after A.A., but which address other
problems, or in any other non–A.A. context, does not imply otherwise.

Contents

Illustrations

Preface

This project and the people upon whom it is based have been part of my life for over fifteen years now. It has been both an exciting and a daunting task to translate the wealth of ethnographic data that I have gathered into published form. Conducting field research in Native North America can be a difficult undertaking for a non-Native anthropologist, and in coming to terms with these challenges I find as I write that I rely more heavily on material gathered through formal interviews than that from the informal flow of participant observation. Each type of information, however, shapes the other, in my thinking.

I am grateful to the Woodrow Wilson Foundation, the Howell Foundation, Wellesley College, the University of California at San Diego, and the University of Iowa for funding various phases of my research to date at Northern Cheyenne. Many thanks are due to the editors, reviewers, and staff at the University of Arizona Press, who have been essential in bringing this book into being.

Some material presented in part II was previously published in Prussing (2007) and Prussing (2008), and sections of part III also appeared in Prussing (2008).

Several different orthographic conventions for Cheyenne have been introduced since the first written form for the language was developed in the late 1800s. I have generally followed the conventions of a dictionary produced by the Northern Cheyenne Title VII Bilingual Education Program in 1976 but have substituted the more accessible "?" for the Latin character used therein to represent a glottal stop.

Many friends and colleagues have provided much-appreciated intellectual insight and moral support through the various stages of this project's development. F. G. Bailey has been an invaluable mentor to me in learning about both anthropology and writing (though I take full responsibility for any awkward prose that appears here). Many thanks are due to Suzanne Brenner, Stephen E. Cornell, Ross Frank, Martha Lampland, and

Michael Meeker for their advice and support during my years at UCSD. I want to express special thanks to Heather Claussen, Elisa J. Sobo, Nancy Hynes, Axel Aubrun, and Andrew Brown for years of friendship and conversation that have helped to shape my work as an anthropologist, as well as to members of the ad hoc writer's support group that coalesced at UCSD in the late 1990s (including Leila Madge, Julia Offen, Jason James, Jeffrey Bass, Lisa Rosen, Tom Brown, Julie Pokrandt, and Andrew Willford). Intermittent but ongoing conversations with Carol Ward and David Wilson, with their extensive research experience and friendships on the Northern Cheyenne Reservation, have enriched my work and life. As time has passed, I have been fortunate to find new colleagues, such as Joe Gone, doing fascinating work on mental health issues in Native North America. I am also deeply grateful to colleagues at the University of Iowa who have provided an essential combination of intellectual insight and practical advice during the writing of this book, including Rudi Colloredo-Mansfeld, Laurie Graham, and Mike Chibnik. Very special thanks are also due to Ellen Lewin, who graciously read a draft of the entire manuscript and provided me with an invaluable combination of constructive criticism and affirmation when I faced a moment of crisis.

I sincerely thank my parents, John and Laurel Prussing, for their continued support and interest through all the years of this project. My husband, Dan McRoberts, and our two sons have welcomed my Northern Cheyenne friends and experiences as part of their own lives. With their help I hope to continue moving among my roles as wife, mother, researcher, teacher, and writer with humor and, I hope, some degree of grace.

Finally, I express my deepest thanks to the numerous Northern Cheyenne community members who lent their time to participate in this project and/or to provide me with feedback on drafts of the various publications that have resulted. I hope that I have accurately represented their perspectives and experiences here, and effectively enabled others to appreciate and learn from them. Any remaining errors are my own.

All proceeds from sales of this book will be donated to the Northern Cheyenne Tribal Health Services.

White Man's Water

1
Introduction: Sobriety and Subjectivity in Local Worlds

I must have been 14 the first time I drank alcohol. It was good, we had fun, nothing happened. There were more girls than boys. They would get an older person to go buy it. I really didn't get into drinking, though—maybe once in a while pitch in for beer, go to that guy's [the local bootlegger] and go get beer. And we goofed off, sang and danced. But next day I didn't like the feeling—like, sick to my stomach, or have to throw up. But it seemed like, it wasn't—it wasn't really that bad, you know, like now. (Josephine,[1] born 1930s)

[When we would go to town,] most of my time was spent waiting for [my parents] in bars. And my diet used to be sardines, and crackers, and orange or grape pop, and barbeque potato chips. To this day I cannot drink or even eat none of that stuff. [We would] sit on the car, and I remember it used to be hotter than hell, 100 degrees, and I used to be sitting outside, waiting 'til the bars closed. I don't even remember them coming out to check on us. . . . I came to a point where I didn't want to go home [from boarding school], 'cause I knew I'd come home and they'd have hangovers, and they'd be in bad moods, or you know it was that typical drunk talk, broken promises stuff. And I just got tired of that, and knew better, so I just—I think it forced me to grow up pretty fast. (Becky, born 1950s)

Tribal members born before and after 1950 encountered markedly different worlds on the Northern Cheyenne Reservation in southeastern Montana. Major midcentury changes included a renewed entrenchment of widespread poverty, a marked rise in social diversity among tribal members, and a sharp increase in alcohol use throughout the community. In constructing narratives about how these changes have impacted their personal and collective well-being, contemporary Northern Cheyennes weave together a variety of narrative themes and forms, some of which are visible in the brief excerpts from Josephine and Becky above.

Josephine portrays alcohol in her adolescence as an occasional and fairly benign presence, producing fun times and only a few unpleasant physical aftereffects. She explicitly minimizes the problems that drinking generated then compared to the present ("not like now"). While briefly implicating possible causes (e.g., gender roles and relations, in noting that there were "more girls than boys"), her rhetorical emphasis here is not to explain so much as to describe how alcohol's negative impact grew over her lifetime. Having grown up two decades later, in contrast, Becky describes drinking as pervasive in her childhood experiences. She positions alcohol as the cause of painful episodes of parental neglect in her childhood and emphasizes the emotional dimensions of her resulting experiences of alienation and abandonment. Echoes of addiction/recovery discourse derived from the Twelve Steps of Alcoholics Anonymous are visible in Becky's portrait of how the family dynamics of alcoholism (e.g., "typical drunk talk") produced this emotional pain, and were detrimental to her personal development ("forced me to grow up pretty fast").

Attending closely to the personal narratives about alcohol produced by Josephine, Becky, and other Northern Cheyenne community members reveals how accounts of subjective experience take shape within a distinctive local cultural landscape—and reflect its diversity and debate. In constructing a decline from a past era, for example, Josephine's narrative holds striking similarities to prominent local rhetorical conventions for understanding threats to Cheyenne well-being in terms of the historical changes wrought by colonization. An idiom of "forgetting" what one did or should know about how to be Cheyenne dominates such accounts. While these local rhetorical frameworks bear superficial similarities to the narratives of loss that characterize many non-Native accounts of indigenous peoples' histories in the United States, they are shaped by a distinctly local set of moral priorities, political goals, and cultural resources. For example, such local commentary imbues meaning and power in Cheyenne action, affirms the importance of maintaining cultural distinctiveness from mainstream U.S. society, and draws upon the rhetorical features set forth in key local traditions of prophecy.

Narratives like Becky's that make use of Twelve Step terms and concepts are also situated within this localized cultural world. Most do not simply recapitulate Twelve Step vocabulary and concepts wholesale, but rather engage in a selective and creative process of appropriation

that variably acknowledges, challenges, and employs the locally prominent rhetorical conventions noted above. A central idiom that attributes
drinking to "cycles" of psychological pain permeates such narratives, a
rhetorical tool drawn directly from Twelve Step approaches to recovery. Yet many who use it also explicitly address colonialism as a cause
of drinking and identify distinctively local cultural resources such as
Cheyenne spiritual practices as essential for sustained sobriety.

Efforts to use Cheyenne spiritual practices can spark considerable
debate, however, highlighting how the multiple local cultural meanings that surround alcohol circulate and produce social consequences
on the reservation. For example, by the 1990s a number of Northern
Cheyenne women were actively weaving together elements of Twelve
Step approaches with efforts to learn and revitalize Cheyenne ritual practices. These efforts elicited a controversial mix of support and criticism
from the broader reservation community, highlighting the broader political dynamics that surround social and cultural change "on the rez." As
such, the Twelve Steps not only are used in culturally distinctive ways at
Northern Cheyenne but also have distinctively localized consequences.

The ethnographic findings that I present here attend to the cultural
shaping of personal narratives, to the politics of how these perspectives
interact in local social life, and to the consequences that these processes
have for individuals seeking sobriety, in order to highlight the variable ways in which Northern Cheyenne community members experience alcohol-related problems and conceptualize the transformation
from drinking to sobriety. Differences in age, gender, family, education,
employment, and other factors for example have produced multiple subjectivities among community members, or modes of perception, interpretation, motivation, and action that are personal but nonetheless culturally patterned and socially influenced (Biehl et al. 2007). At Northern
Cheyenne, what have resulted are debates over how to construct identity,
self and self-transformation, emotional experience and expression, and
social authority, and these shape efforts to define and address alcohol-
related health problems. Moves to achieve and/or promote sobriety elicit
diverse and often conflicting responses among community members,
and the ongoing social interactions among individuals and groups who
hold different perspectives on alcohol contribute new layers of meaning
to any therapeutic approach that is introduced on the reservation.

Effective services for alcohol-related health problems on the reservation need to respond to this diversity. During the period 1994–2005,

the capacity of local substance abuse services to respond to these complexities was limited, shaped in part by the distinctive political economy of federally funded health services on the reservation that continually positioned Twelve Step vocabulary, concepts, and practices as the default approach to supporting sobriety. Since the 1950s, programs based on the Twelve Steps have been institutionalized in federally funded health services in Native American communities such as Northern Cheyenne. Yet Northern Cheyenne community members frequently criticize these services for their lack of fit with prevalent local definitions of normal and pathological drinking, conventions for social interaction, and ethnopsychological constructions of person and emotion (see also Spicer 2001). Critics frequently cite quitting on one's own as a preferable alternative. The Northern Cheyenne community does not have formalized local therapeutic systems that can easily be institutionalized as alternatives for promoting sobriety, however. Efforts to craft more culturally appropriate methods for promoting and sustaining sobriety are instead taking shape at a grassroots level. Yet the stipulations of funding and regulatory agencies place ongoing material and discursive pressures on health services to construct "one size fits all" solutions. Examining how illustrates the extent to which implementing local control of health services remains difficult in communities like Northern Cheyenne, despite unprecedented gains in Native American capacities for medical self-determination in recent decades (Adams 2000; Noren et al. 1998).

In calling for more culturally appropriate alcohol services, the story that I tell here also describes the actions that Northern Cheyenne community members are taking to adapt available services to better fit local needs. Attending to their efforts can yield insights into how local cultural distinctiveness persists at Northern Cheyenne after generations of colonization and under globalized pressures in mental health services. Despite widespread criticism, for example, a heterogeneous array of adults and youth at Northern Cheyenne do engage Twelve Step ideas and practices, often modifying them to better fit the local realities of their lives and experiences. Why, and for whom, do the Twelve Steps hold appeal on the reservation? How are they used in ways that reflect the local cultural landscape, including its key features of diversity and debate?

To answer these questions I conducted participant observation in a variety of contexts on the Northern Cheyenne Reservation, and individual interviews with community members, during an initial three-year stay (1994–97), an extended follow-up visit in 2005, and numerous shorter visits in between. The politics of gender clearly play a key role in the cultural politics that surround sobriety at Northern Cheyenne. While a number of Northern Cheyenne men certainly make use of Twelve Step resources, staff at the reservation's addiction recovery program report that between the 1970s and 1990s, the male-to-female ratio of their clients shifted from approximately 3:1 to 1:1.5. By the 1990s women had become highly visible in attending and leading community-based Twelve Step meetings, and in organizing public workshops about recovery-related topics.

The role of gender in shaping the appeal of the Twelve Steps is clearly situated among other factors, however, since the overwhelming majority of women involved in these activities were born in the 1950s or later. Many of these women expressed criticism of core Twelve Step concepts (such as "alcoholism") and departed from conventional Twelve Step practices (e.g., regularly attending meetings). A fuller explanation of the local social life of the Twelve Steps at Northern Cheyenne therefore needs to account for the generational differences among women, and for the selective and creative dimensions of how younger generations of women are making use of Twelve Step approaches. Such an explanation also needs to address the fact that women's efforts to adapt Twelve Step approaches for local use have included integrating them with efforts to revitalize local spiritual traditions, and associated controversies.

A detailed ethnographic study of these questions responds to recent calls in medical and psychological anthropology for "deeper depictions of the local" (Kleinman and Kleinman 1997:19), to illuminate how globalized discourses about suffering and healing can reverberate through the intertwining realms of cultural representations, social experience, and subjectivity within localized communities. Such calls reflect anthropology's growing efforts to better link the interpretations, motivations, and actions of social actors to the political-economic landscape of constraints and opportunities that they inhabit. In working to further integrate individual experiences into contemporary social theory, and to better document the lived realities of "personalizing culture resources" (Parish 2008:188), psychological anthropologists are increasingly examining how historical conditions such as colonialism and its ongoing legacies of social inequality are shaping cultural constructions of emotion and morality—and how these in turn are incorporated into individual experiences of social life, modes of self-expression, and motivation (Biehl et al. 2007; Desjarlais and O'Nell 2000; M. Good et al. 2008).

The notion of a complex thinking and feeling actor, with multiple and sometimes conflicting motivations, distinguishes approaches to subjectivity in psychological anthropology from the emphasis on the production of subject positions through discourse in much contemporary social theory (Brenneis 2000; B. Good et al. 2008).

Recent ethnographic works in Native North America have offered productive models for how to attend to both the psychological and the sociopolitical dimensions of talk, appreciating how distinctive local meanings and debates surrounding "tradition," for example, can inform the ways in which self-transformation is expressed and then responded to by socially significant others. In her work about depression in the Flathead Reservation community, O'Nell (1996) documents the contested nature of identity claims among tribal members with diverse social backgrounds and historical experiences, and how these are oriented by a dominant conceptualization of tradition that is variously deployed to include or exclude individuals and/or their particular claims to community membership. Csordas and colleagues (Csordas 1999; Dole and Csordas 2003), examining religious healing on the Navajo Reservation, describe how the concept of tradition organizes experiences and expressions of identity, and how the meanings attributed to tradition may vary by generation. These portraits also demonstrate how attending to positioning in social structure and to the politics of talk need not exclude consideration of psychological realities. For Native North American contexts, they specifically highlight the potential semantic overlap between "tradition" and "culture," and how this may inform psychological experience and its representation differently for different sectors of a community. Here I extend these considerations into an analysis of drinking and sobriety and emphasize an additional dimension of gender. While the gendered dimensions of subjectivity are cogently addressed in numerous works about the cultural situatedness of psychological experience (e.g., Abu-Lughod 1986; Behar 2003; Borovoy 2005), to date these have rarely been emphasized in studies of Native North American drinking (cf. Fast 2002) or explicitly linked to the localized politics that can surround mental health services in contemporary Native communities.

The question of whether Twelve Step approaches help Northern Cheyenne community members to effectively abstain from or reduce their substance use is certainly an important one. Yet, to fully answer it requires first asking broader questions about how these approaches are culturally and socially situated in a local context. Doing so affirms the need for indigenous self-determination in health care and considers how the special insights afforded by ethnographic research might be used to improve the cultural appropriateness of health services.

"Culture" in "Culturally Appropriate" Alcohol Services

Closer examination of how Northern Cheyenne community members use and respond to others' use of Twelve Step approaches to sobriety highlights how these approaches variably alienate and appeal to reservation residents. To say that the socially patterned appeal of the Twelve Steps at Northern Cheyenne is locally distinctive is not to say that it is entirely unique, however. Alienation from Twelve Step concepts and practices is not limited to Native North America (Kasl 1992; Madsen 1974; Peele 1989). The special appeal of the Twelve Steps and related "pop" psychologies to younger generations (Irvine 1999) and to women (Simonds 1992) also extends beyond the Northern Cheyenne Reservation, shaped by broader historical shifts in U.S. cultural mores and social institutions by the late twentieth century. Moreover, Twelve Step concepts and practices have remained prominent in substance abuse treatment centers and programs throughout the United States since the 1950s, despite ongoing criticism and efforts to implement more secular, culturally appropriate, and/ or evidence-based alternatives (White 1998). Yet conditions at Northern Cheyenne illuminate distinctive local meanings and social consequences of Twelve Step approaches to sobriety, as well as the special challenges of providing culturally appropriate alcohol services on the reservation.

Efforts to better recognize and accommodate cultural differences have become a key priority in U.S. health care in recent decades. Federal agencies such as the Office of Minority Health and the Health Resources and Services Administration now position improving "cultural competence" among their central goals, and health initiatives by influential private foundations such as the Commonwealth Fund, Kaiser Family Foundation, and Robert Wood Johnson Foundation also widely reference this concept. These concerns have sparked special interest among mental health professionals, visible in the "Mental Health: Culture, Race and Ethnicity" (Department of Health and Human Services 2001) supplement to the broader 1999 mental health report of the Surgeon General.

To date, anthropological perspectives have figured rather unevenly in these efforts. Anthropologists generally view alcohol, for example, as a culturally constructed substance that is often subject to regulation by states and other governing bodies but is ultimately perceived, used, and in some cases avoided within localized social structures and worlds of meaning (Douglas 1987; Heath 2000; Marshall 1979). These local cultural worlds are historically situated and subject to change (Eber 2000; Marshall and Marshall 1990). From this perspective, distinctions between normal and pathological alcohol use vary significantly by time, place, and person. Moreover, therapeutic transformations from drinking to sobriety (Bezdek and Spicer 2006; Eber 2000; Kunitz and Levy 1994; Marshall and Marshall 1990; Quintero 2000; Spicer 2001) are culturally mediated shifts in behavior and subjective experience that may require considerable negotiation with socially significant others.

Anthropology's focus on variability holds a rather tense relationship with the more widely known perspectives in the clinical practices of psychiatry and psychology and the prevention campaigns of public health, which emphasize universalizing definitions of mental health problems and interventions that transcend such local particulars (Lee and Kleinman 2007; Mezzich et al. 1999). Even when efforts are made to accommodate cultural differences in mental health services, they often employ essentializing logics through understanding "culture" as a clearly definable set of beliefs and practices that are generally shared by a given community. For example, the "Mental Health: Culture, Race and Ethnicity" supplement noted above laudably discusses how culturally specific assumptions and priorities shape the perceptions and actions of both clinicians and patients, and includes input from anthropologists (Good and Good 2003). Yet it also reflects ongoing debate about how to conceptualize and measure cultural influences on mental health (Good and Good 2003), and includes extended descriptions of specific beliefs and practices that could be read as stereotypes of how particular ethnic groups think and act. Anthropological theory increasingly emphasizes how "culture" is an arena of contested meanings and debate (Ortner 2006), however, and research in medical anthropology documents how multiple and contested understandings, priorities, and perspectives within cultural communities can affect how health conditions are experienced and resources utilized (Hahn 1999; Lindenbaum and Lock 1993; Nichter and Lock 2002). Medical anthropologists have been especially critical of how efforts toward cultural competence in biomedicine, while clearly necessary, all too often end up reproducing rather than moving beyond static views of "culture" in representing groups by ethnicity, race, language, or other perceived features (Kleinman and Benson 2006; Taylor 2003).

Such stereotyping logics are especially likely to accompany health behaviors that tend to provoke intense moral discourse in the United States, such as alcohol and drug use. Such logics function even more vigorously when such behaviors are practiced by people whose social identities also subject them to enhanced moral scrutiny.

Ambivalent views of alcohol have an especially lengthy history in the United States. The circulation of negative ideas about drinking seems to have widened as nineteenth-century industrialization articulated new standards of productivity and respectability. People who drank habitually or to excess, by these new standards, were far more likely to be perceived as morally degenerate or medically diseased (McDonald 1994). The American Temperance Movement of the nineteenth century helped to popularize these ideas, linking sobriety to popular Protestant notions of thrift and hard work (Gusfield 1986). Through the twentieth century, public policies such as Prohibition in the 1920s, public health campaigns about the detrimental effects of alcohol use (Peele 1993), the institutionalization of medical research about problematic drinking with the establishment of the National Institute on Alcohol Abuse and Alcoholism, and activism by groups like Mothers Against Drunk Driving (Marshall and Oleson 1996) have continued to reflect and arguably perpetuate morally charged perspectives on the pathological aspects of alcohol use. These perspectives coexist with competing views that link alcohol use to good times, recreation, and sexual attractiveness, however. Singer (2008) compellingly demonstrates how the U.S. alcohol industry (and similarly, the tobacco and prescription drug industries) strategically responds to moral and scientific claims about the adverse consequences of its products in order to maintain and expand its markets. These polarized interpretations leave limited room for clear discussions of either the detrimental consequences or the benefits of alcohol use, and visibly conflict with anthropology's multifaceted and open-ended perspective on drinking.

These tendencies to rely on oversimplified and morally charged stereotypes are intensified when attention turns to drinking by social groups that are already subject to special moral monitoring. Armstrong (2003) demonstrates how morally vested cultural assumptions about motherhood in the late twentieth century have intersected with long-standing cultural themes of ambivalence about alcohol use in North America. The result has been the production and circulation of intense pejorative stereotypes of women who drink during pregnancy, and an array of vigorous public health information campaigns and legal consequences in the

United States that, many argue, actually interfere with effective prevention efforts (see Oaks 2001 for a similar argument about tobacco use during pregnancy). Similar moral discourse and medico-legal responses are applied to alcohol and other drug use by stigmatized groups such as people in poverty (Singer 2008) or members of minoritized racial and ethnic groups (Krauss 1991). Stereotyped imagery and assumptions about "drunken Indians" are especially entrenched in the United States and pose special challenges for appreciating the diversity of experiences with drinking and sobriety that actually occur among Native North Americans.

From "Indian Drinking" to "White Man's Water"

Stereotypes about the universality and severity of "Indian drinking" remain hugely popular in North America, despite strong challenges from decades of social scientific research. Attending to the diverse local meanings and practices that surround alcohol at Northern Cheyenne, and situating these local perceptions and debates within a historical context, constructively disrupts such popular perceptions. Indeed, a key Cheyenne term for alcohol (*vé?ho?e-mahpe*) translates as "white man's water," reflecting local perceptions of how colonization, race, and alcohol use are inextricably intertwined. Commentary about contemporary reservation problems at Northern Cheyenne often reflects prominent local rhetorical conventions for discussing the nature and scope of threats to collective well-being, yet these are used in very different ways by different community members. Listening closely to commentary about alcohol highlights how these ongoing localized politics socially pattern the appeal of particular therapeutic resources like the Twelve Steps.

These cultural complexities are not well known to most North Americans. Instead, popular representations of Native peoples continue to reflect and perpetuate a long-standing colonial narrative that accommodates moral ambivalence about Euro-American colonization while ultimately justifying it. Classic early works in Native American studies (Berkhofer 1978; Dippie 1982) emphasize how, when constructed through the image of the Noble Savage, popular colonial narratives can sentimentalize and mourn the losses experienced by Native peoples. By portraying Native peoples as degraded heathens, however, the same basic narrative can be used to celebrate their demise through death or assimilation. In either case, the overall effect is to reinforce perceptions of a fundamental difference between Native and non-Native. Kessler (1996) emphasizes how gender has always shaped this colonial narrative, noting how key images of Native women integrated a broader narrative of manifest destiny with common American cultural stereotypes of women (e.g., as wife, mother, whore, siren, witch), and offered further justification for establishing U.S. colonial control over Native lands and bodies (see also Smith 2005).

Popular stereotypes about Native peoples and alcohol echo these colonial storylines by also positioning Native peoples at the moral margins of the social order in the United States. Berkhofer (1978) directly references alcohol in an example of how "reservation Indians" have been constructed within the morally corrupt liminal space between the long-standing colonial constructs of "civilization" and "Indianness": "this degraded, often drunken, Indian . . . living as neither an assimilated White nor an Indian of the classic image, and therefore neither noble nor wildly savage but always scorned, the degraded Indian exhibited the vices of both societies in the opinion of White observers" (1978:30).

While popular portrayals of Native American women's drinking are limited, these especially emphasize such themes of tragedy and pathology. Michael Dorris's best-selling account of adopting a Lakota child with fetal alcohol syndrome, or FAS (1990), offers a well-known example. While FAS is a serious problem that certainly deserves close attention, Dorris's portrait echoes the gendered assumptions and maternal–fetal conflict perspective on pregnancy highlighted by Armstrong's analysis (see above) and ultimately calls for the criminalization of Native women's drinking while pregnant. Yet this call distorts the fact that most Native women's drinking does not result in FAS, and it overlooks how legal penalties are likely to alienate women from seeking help. Better understanding of the broader scope of Native women's reasons for starting and stopping drinking is also essential to preventing the adverse effects of alcohol. These effects are by no means limited to pregnancy but include many points in a woman's life and that of her family and community.

Recent social theory offers useful tools for considering the multiple dimensions of Northern Cheyenne women's experiences living on a reservation, and for responding to both personal and collective problems with alcohol there. Insights from practice theory (Bourdieu 1990; Holland and Leander 2004; Ortner 2006) illuminate how the lived experiences, activities, and goals of social actors are diversely shaped by variable social positioning from cultural and historical forces. Critical theory (Fabian 1991; Scheper-Hughes 1992; Singer and Baer 1995) complements this perspective by examining what power relations are served by over-looking these complexities and relying instead on essentializing categories and logics. Feminist works in medical anthropology especially attend to the multiple cultural meanings of health-related conditions (e.g., Van Hollen 2003) and medical technologies (e.g., Rapp 1999), and to the diverse and often strategic practices that result among those who encounter them (e.g., Lock and Kaufert 1998).

Attention to how power inequalities shape cultural meanings and social practices is also central to the question of how and why the reservation's primary institutionalized program to support sobriety has remained oriented around the Twelve Steps, despite widespread local criticism and clear evidence of ongoing grassroots efforts toward alternatives. Yet very little ethnographic work has been done about Twelve Step approaches to sobriety in Native American communities. Indeed, with several important exceptions, ethnographic research about alcohol has largely overlooked the rising global popularity of Twelve Step approaches to sobriety.

Twelve Step Therapies: Discourse and Practice

The Twelve Steps arose with the emergence of Alcoholics Anonymous in the United States in the 1930s and posited a universalized "disease model" of alcohol addiction (i.e., alcoholism). In its widespread literature, A.A. defines alcoholism as a "progressive, incurable, and fatal" disease that can be managed with a systematic therapeutic program centered on attending meetings to talk with other alcoholics about past and present experiences (Alcoholics Anonymous 2002). This disease model construes alcoholism as a fundamental disorder in the coherence and stability of the self, generating troubling emotions (anger, blame, self-pity) that one attempts to avoid or manage through drunkenness (Denzin 1987). Sobriety is achieved by comprehensive psychological reorientation, self-transformation through a Twelve Step program of personal growth. The series of steps (first, six; later expanded to twelve) was developed by A.A. founders in the decade after the group was founded. This therapeutic approach is explicitly not concerned with the psychological causes of addiction problems but is grounded in the idea that behavior change will itself lead to psychological change (White 1998). A.A. therefore casts a person's relationship with alcohol itself as the cause of problems and

The Twelve Steps of Alcoholics Anonymous

1. We admitted we were powerless over alcohol---that our lives had become unmanageable.
2. Came to believe that a Power greater than ourselves could restore us to sanity.
3. Made a decision to turn our will and our lives over to the care of God *as we understood Him*.
4. Made a searching and fearless moral inventory of ourselves.
5. Admitted to God, to ourselves, and to another human being the exact nature of our wrongs.
6. Were entirely ready to have God remove all these defects of character.
7. Humbly asked Him to remove our shortcomings.
8. Made a list of all persons we had harmed, and became willing to make amends to them all.
9. Made direct amends to such people wherever possible, except when to do so would injure them or others.
10. Continued to take personal inventory and when we were wrong promptly admitted it.
11. Sought through prayer and meditation to improve our conscious contact with God, *as we understood Him*, praying only for knowledge of His will for us and the power to carry that out.
12. Having had a spiritual awakening as the result of these Steps, we tried to carry this message to alcoholics, and to practice these principles in all our affairs.

Figure 1. The Twelve Steps. Reprinted with permission of Alcoholics Anonymous World Services, Inc.

frames this relationship as permanent through encouraging members to identify themselves as "alcoholics."

The first step involves overcoming denial that one's drinking is out of control and causing negative consequences by "admitting powerlessness" over alcohol (Alcoholics Anonymous 2002). Key subsequent steps involve countering the self-centeredness of alcoholism by embracing the concept of a power greater than oneself (whether God or another higher power), thereby reorienting and expanding one's psychosocial world. Self-reflection about one's need to improve (see step 4) and continuing to "take personal inventory" (see step 10) by reflecting upon and evaluating one's behavior are seen as essential to maintaining this focus. Continuing to meet with other alcoholics to share experiences supports this broader process, on the theory that maintaining sobriety is a lifelong process requiring constant reminders that being an alcoholic includes an ongoing tendency to relapse into past psychological and/or behavioral patterns. The role of talk in therapeutic transformation is heavily emphasized here, grounded in notions that if one does not talk about painful experiences, then one cannot work through them, manage them, and limit their power over one's thoughts, feelings, and actions.

As Cain (1991), Antze (1987), Swora (2001), and others have noted, the Twelve Steps provide a symbolic system and set of narrative templates that participants learn and reproduce in a highly conventionalized style of self-expression that is monitored and evaluated by other participants. These stylized practices, along with the spiritual focus and reliance on a higher power encoded within the Twelve Steps, have been criticized for decades for alienating many who seek or need help for their troubling involvements with alcohol (Kasl 1992; Madsen 1974; White 1998). More recently, critics have emphasized that scientific evidence is lacking not only for the assumptions about addiction and recovery within Twelve Step therapies but also for their efficacy (Fingarette 1989; Miller 2008; Peele 1989). Yet despite ongoing criticism, Twelve Step ideas and practices became hugely influential in both public policy and addiction treatment in North America between the 1940s and 1980s (White 1998), including Native North American mental health programs (Gone 2008). One of the most prominent therapeutic models for treating alcohol abuse in the United States arose at various sites in Minnesota starting in the 1950s.

As White (1998) describes, the emergence of this "Minnesota Model" for alcohol treatment expressly aimed to integrate ideas and practices from the self-help groups of Alcoholics Anonymous with clinical treatment for alcohol addiction. From the 1950s through the 1970s this approach melded multiple therapeutic disciplines together under a Twelve Step–oriented framework. Twelve Step ideas are clearly visible in how it casts alcoholism as incurable and progressive but manageable, and emphasizes the therapeutic importance of clients (a) working with a counselor who is ideally a recovering alcoholic with whom they can share experiences, and (b) attending group meetings to exchange experiences with other clients. Effective intervention involves a multidisciplinary team and an individualized treatment plan, with the express goal of completing the first five of the Twelve Steps while in treatment and then continuing to receive ongoing support afterward through attending Twelve Step meetings (Hazelden 2010). Hazelden in Center City, Minnesota, is perhaps the premier treatment center that developed and adopted this approach, heavily influencing alcohol treatment efforts throughout the United States by serving as a key site for interns and trainees from the growing networks for addiction research and treatment that had formed between the 1940s and 1960s (e.g., new professional training programs, research and clinical conferences, summer schools, and national organizations), and also by producing and disseminating numerous publications about recovery (White 1998).

Twelve Step ideas and practices not only became mainstays of formal treatment programs for addiction in the United States but also expanded their grassroots base in the decades following the 1930s. For example, the scope of Twelve Step programs successively expanded beyond A.A.'s initial focus on a predominantly white and male membership whose central problem was drinking. "Specialty A.A. meetings" emerged to focus on the special needs of populations defined by gender, age, or ethnicity, as well as a diverse array of other social categories such as "gays and lesbians, doctors, those with 'double troubles' (dual diagnoses), the poly-addicted, non-smokers, newcomers, pilots, old-timers, agnostics, and bikers" (White 1998:162). By the 1960s and 1970s Twelve Step groups had also formed for people who were not alcoholics themselves but who were nevertheless affected by alcoholism in their families as spouses (Al-Anon) and children (Alateen) (Irvine 1999). By the 1970s, the rise of family systems theory in American psychotherapy offered further support for conceptualizing addiction as a dysfunction in interpersonal relationships that can be passed across generations. By the 1980s, Adult Children of Alcoholics (ACOA) groups arose to address the stunting of emotional life and distortion of social relationships theorized to result as families develop "rules" to accommodate an active alcoholic (e.g., "Don't talk, don't trust, don't feel" [Black 2001:33]). ACOA holds that children of alcoholics are predisposed to seek out mates and situations that replicate these patterns, recapitulating destructive "cycles" over time. Recovery involves attending ACOA meetings and working a Twelve Step program that helps one to "detach" from people and situations that elicit these cycles, as well as to get in touch with one's "inner child" to heal the pain of early experiences of abandonment, neglect, and abuse.

By this era too, the concept of "codependency" further expanded the scope of behaviors and experiences interpretable as manifestations of "addiction." By its terms, personal unhappiness and unfulfilling relationships do not require growing up with an addict in the family but simply within a "dysfunctional" family and/or society. Casting codependency as a "master addiction" (Irvine 1999:7), proponents broadened the scope of potentially "addictive" behaviors to include not only drinking but also eating, gambling, sex, smoking, shopping, and working as potential ways that codependent individuals cope with the emotional pain associated with their excessive investment in the thoughts, feelings, and responses of others. As with other addictions, recovery from codependency involves working a therapeutic Twelve Step program centered on attending Codependents Anonymous (CoDA) meetings. Perhaps due to its breadth and ambiguity (Kaminer 1992; White 1998), the construct of codependency rapidly became a popular and accessible discursive framework for articulating self and suffering in the United States (Irvine 1999), dominating book sales and talk shows and fueling a boom in treatment centers, workshops, and organizations.

The contemporary addiction/recovery industry in the United States can be read as the consumer capitalist permutation of a much longer-standing American cultural preoccupation with self-help and self-improvement. A.A.'s distinctively Anglo-American flavor is evident in how Twelve Step concepts and practices are firmly grounded within broader Protestant traditions, including an emphasis on self-control, themes of conversion and surrender, and the central role of personal testimony, and through being voluntary and individual (rather than coerced by hierarchical authority) (Brandes 2002; Marshall and Marshall 1990). Arguably, Twelve Step approaches also reflect a broader contemporary American cultural tendency to define spirituality in psychological terms (Barnes 1998).

Yet Twelve Step approaches have also been influential outside of the United States (Borovoy 2005; Brandes 2002; Makela 1996), as well as among culturally diverse populations within North America. Recent decades have witnessed both grassroots and institutionalized efforts to improve the cultural appropriateness of Twelve Step approaches. These include efforts to attend to: culturally appropriate communication practices (e.g., metaphors, language, rituals, role models); how addiction relates to broader legacies of economic, social, and political disempowerment, with associated critical consciousness of how the focus on humility and surrender to a higher power in A.A.'s conventional formulation of the Twelve Steps may run counter to this aim; and the potential utility of locally distinctive support systems for sobriety (White 1998). Versions of Twelve Step approaches have been specifically developed by and for Native North Americans, for example, through local modifications (Coyhis and White 2002; Jilek-Aall 1981), as well as through the development and dissemination of models through federal agencies. By the 1990s, organizations explicitly based on Twelve Step concepts such the National Association for Native American Children of Alcoholics (NANACOA 2005) were active, as were nonprofit support organizations such as White Bison, Inc., which advocates sobriety in a larger project of Native wellness ("wellbriety") through cultural revitalization (Coyhis and White 2002). A genre of recovery books specific to Native Americans emerged from a variety of publishers (e.g., Holmes and McPeek 1988).⁷ A mid-1980s film that was widely disseminated among both Native American communities and cross-cultural alcohol researchers, *The Honour of All,* features A.A. as a key factor in the story of a British Columbian community's radical achievement of near universal sobriety (Lucas 1985).

During this era, the federal Center for Substance Abuse Prevention (Substance Abuse and Mental Health Administration 2005) also developed a "Gathering of Native Americans" (GONA) prevention education curriculum, which served as the foundation for several community workshops for recovery that I attended on the reservation. GONA's approach emphasized the conceptual framework popularized in 1990s Native American health scholarship (e.g., Duran and Duran 1995) that the historical trauma of colonization had multifaceted cultural, psychological, and spiritual consequences that are closely intertwined with substance abuse and other mental health problems among contemporary Native peoples.

Strikingly few ethnographic studies have examined the impact of Twelve Step approaches to recovery in Native North America, however. Commentary about the poor cultural fit of Twelve Step concepts and practices within Native communities (Heath 1983; Spicer 2001) has implied that its presence and impact are limited. Yet other studies describe its significance for at least some communities or population sectors. Baird-Olsen and Ward (2000), for example, document how A.A. is utilized by some women on the Northern Cheyenne and Fort Peck reservations in Montana, in their larger portrait of the dynamic relationships between Christian churches and Native spiritual practices in these two communities during the 1990s.

Indeed, despite its widespread and multifaceted influence on both popular and clinical discourses and practices surrounding alcohol and other substances in numerous cultural settings, relatively few anthropological studies examine Alcoholics Anonymous and related permutations of the Twelve Steps (cf. Quintero and Nichter 1996). A handful of ethnographic studies have examined the efficacy of symbols, narrative strategies, and community support that A.A. employs to transform cognitive and affective experience (Antze 1987; Bateson 1972; Cain 1991; Madsen 1974; Rodin 1985; Sadler 1979; Swora 2001; Wilcox 1998). Many draw parallels to healing practices in other cultural contexts, such as cults of affliction (Antze 1987; Madsen 1979; Sadler 1979; Swora 2001); and several have also specifically focused on better specifying the relationships between biological and sociocultural dimensions of problematic drinking (Madsen 1979; Rodin 1985). Some have also examined how A.A. and related addiction/recovery approaches are shaped by distinctive cultural purposes when used outside of Anglo-America (e.g., Borovoy 2005; Brandes 2002; Jilek-Aall 1981; Makela 1996), documenting the importance of cross-cultural continuities as well as localized cultural modifications of these approaches.[3] Such work has clear potential to help improve alcohol-related health services and raises theoretical questions about subjective experience, power, and therapeutic transformation that are of broader interest within medical anthropology.

For indigenous communities specifically, the ways in which Twelve Step approaches have often become institutionalized through federally funded health service systems pose further questions about the ongoing tensions among ongoing regional, national, and international efforts to promote greater local control over health services.

Indigenous Self-Determination in Health: Local Complexities

Following decades of activism, a new generation of health programs in New Zealand, Canada, Australia, the United States, and elsewhere includes active efforts to decolonize health services by better accommodating the cultural worlds of indigenous communities (Davies 2001; Durie 1998; Kelm 2004; Lavoie 2004; Warry 1998). Some Native American communities in the United States have successfully established local control over a variety of health services (Adams 2000; Noren et al. 1998), including alcohol services (Hall 1986). The considerable variation among communities in their historical experiences, population numbers relative to non-Natives in their region, local and regional economic resources, and so forth shapes the feasibility of such efforts. My conversations with numerous indigenous health workers and researchers throughout North America suggest that the difficulties with exerting local control that I witnessed at Northern Cheyenne from 1994 to 2005 are not uncommon. Barriers to indigenous control of health care have deep historical roots in the United States especially. Physician-historian David Jones (2004) offers a cogent analysis of how continuing colonial legacies and entrenched non-Native ambivalence about Native cultural survival in the United States have helped to continually reproduce health inequalities over the course of five centuries, often through haphazard and underfunded health services.

Services for sobriety that are genuinely culturally appropriate, for instance, would effectively engage prevalent local modes of understanding both drinking and the behavioral change of sobriety. While the global trend toward recognizing the need for more "culturally competent" health services has permeated the addiction treatment industry (White 1998), barriers remain to incorporating full recognition of the complexities of local cultural contexts into such services. Indeed, the form and impact of such efforts vary in indigenous-controlled health programs. Some incorporate local cultural elements while continuing to emphasize globally prominent therapies such as those derived from the Twelve Steps (e.g., Hall 1986; Weibel-Orlando 1989), while others purposefully assert local cultural ideas and practices as either complementary or alternative therapy (e.g., Brady 1995; Gone 2008). On a material level many of these programs remain partially if not fully federally funded and regulated by non-indigenous accreditation agencies (Kunitz and Levy 1994), and on an ideological level many are structured in response to prevailing therapeutic paradigms in the surrounding non-indigenous society (Gone 2008).

Many ethnographers support greater local community control as a strategy to improve the effectiveness of mental health services in indigenous communities (Kirmayer et al. 2000; O'Nell 2000, 2004). Yet Weibel-Orlando (1989) cautions that anthropologists too easily slip into assuming that indigenous healing approaches are automatically effective, and that programs for Native Americans need to be categorically different from non-Native programs (see also Levy and Kunitz 1974). Brady echoes these concerns in observing how indigenous "culture" is being used to define substance abuse as a simple and straightforward effect of the disruptions of colonization in Australian Aboriginal addiction services, "which seem to valorize an imagined authenticity" (1995:1487) rather than attending to more complex realities—including, Brady suggests, how "traditional" cultural features may in some cases not inhibit but in fact promote the problematic use of substances.

Assertions that indigenous cultural revitalization facilitates recovery can be read as a form of "strategic essentialism" (Guha and Spivak 1988), and as a challenge to popular but pejorative stereotypes about the inevitability of "Indian drinking." Close attention to the example of the complex local politics that surround such claims at Northern Cheyenne helps to illustrate how, whether racist or antiracist in intent, essentializing claims about complex psychological phenomena need to be examined critically.

Setting: Reservation Snapshots

The Northern Cheyenne Reservation includes approximately 450,000 acres of semiarid grassy plains and pine-covered hills in the southeastern corner of Montana. The overwhelming majority of reservation residents are Northern Cheyenne tribal members, with the remainder mostly members of other tribes, and only about 5 percent non-Natives (Ward and Wilson 1989). Many live in the central village of Lame Deer, and others in the smaller settlements of Ashland, Busby, and Birney, while a small number dwell on rural homesteads. Infrequent non-Indian towns dot the landscape surrounding the reservation. With the major exception of Billings, Montana (100 miles to the west of Lame Deer and home to some 80,000), and the smaller cities of Sheridan, Wyoming, to the south and Miles City, Montana, to the northeast, most have populations

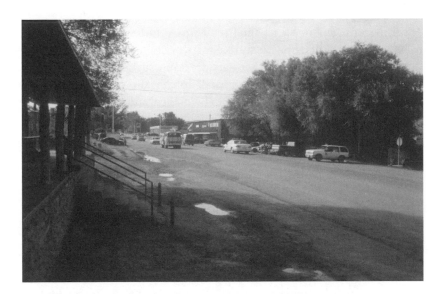

Figure 2. Main street in Lame Deer, Montana. Photo by the author.

of under 3,000. The regional economy is dominated by ranching and mining, with some limited farming. Deer and antelope still roam the countryside, visible from the major highways as well as from the back roads, and hunting is common for both sport and subsistence. The climate runs to extremes, with a short burst of spring followed by many hot and dry weeks of summer, a shorter interlude of cool and occasionally rainy autumn weather, and then months of subzero cold snaps and snow-laden winter days. Compared to the more dramatic river valleys and mountains of the western part of the state, eastern Montana's beauty is understated, resting in its wide horizons, changeable sky, and the subtle seasonal transformations of its greens, browns, and grays.

While the toll that alcohol takes on the well-being of Northern Cheyenne community members may not be easily visible to a casual visitor, it rapidly becomes clear with closer attention. A policy of prohibition is maintained in the tribal legal code, and by the 1990s police efforts did seem to be limiting the visibility of public drunkenness on the reservation itself. Off the reservation Native people were more visible drinking on the sidewalks and street corners in the nearby towns of Ashland and Hardin, or sitting on the logs in the parking lot in front of Jimtown bar (located just a stone's throw from the reservation's northern border).

The impact of alcohol use on the lives of reservation residents is evident in how daily conversations feature efforts to contain the social disruptions created by particular individuals' drinking, such as who will care for their children. Other common topics of conversation include instances of alcohol-related illness, interpersonal violence, and injuries, especially in car accidents. Through kinship ties and social networks, in one way or another, troubling forms of alcohol use clearly touch everyone, even those who have stopped drinking or have never started. Whether or not I formally interviewed them as part of my research, I have found that virtually every Northern Cheyenne person that I have gotten to know well over the past 15 years has lost at least one close family member to alcohol-related illnesses, accidents, or violence.

To better understand the production and circulation of diverse perspectives on alcohol at Northern Cheyenne and how local alcohol services respond to these realities, I participated generally in community life but also focused on especially relevant social arenas like health services—including the Recovery Center alcohol and drug program.

Ethnographic Fieldwork on the Rez

My fieldwork experiences were initially centered in community health programs and public events, and emphasized observation and semistructured interviews. They soon grew to include participant observation of the flow of daily experience on the reservation through an expanding social network centered on several friendships that I was fortunate to develop soon after I arrived. By the second and third years of my initial stay, I focused on more unstructured interviews that allowed further layers of meaning to emerge regarding alcohol, sobriety, and community life.

"Ethnography" has taken on different meanings outside of anthropology and in health research is often considered equivalent to qualitative methods (e.g., conducting interviews) and/or to research that involves patient populations from cultural minority groups (e.g., see Sobo 2009:70–71). Yet within anthropology, hallmarks of ethnographic fieldwork include long-term immersion in a cultural context and learning by participant observation. As I spent time with community health outreach workers on the reservation, for example, many would note landmarks significant to their collective or personal histories as we drove around to visit various patients. On one trip one worker spontaneously pointed out several sites of alcohol-related deaths of her family members, vividly prompting me to realize the extent to which for some community members, the surrounding landscape itself is animated by local histories of alcohol-related violence. I would have never thought or known to ask about this dimension of alcohol's impact on daily lived experience if I had simply conducted interviews with community members.

An effort to cultivate a status that includes elements of both insider and outsider is also key to ethnographic work. While "going native" is not the goal, the process does aim to produce a fundamental transformation in one's cultural skills and resulting perceptions, interpretations, and communication practices. I found myself dreaming differently during and after fieldwork, for example, and reacting to adverse events in ways that increasingly diverged from those of my pre-fieldwork life in ways that sometimes changed relationships with long-standing friends and colleagues. Several years into my work, I was adopted into a Northern Cheyenne family, a means of recognizing my partial status as an "insider." Yet my "outsider" status is still widely evident, visible, for example, in how other community members still tell me negative gossip about my adoptive family members in ways that they would undoubtedly avoid if they viewed me as a true family "insider."

As a research method, ethnography is time-consuming, difficult, and subject to the complexities of gathering information through a social process of interaction. It also often bears the limitations of scope and interpretation that inevitably accompany work by a singular researcher. Its key strengths, however, lie in its capacities to gather rich and multifaceted information about how human experience unfolds in localized contexts. By emphasizing appropriate contextualization and avoiding the "immodest claims" (Farmer 1999:23) of overstating one's conclusions, ethnographic work can significantly improve the validity of research findings.

Social inequalities between ethnographers and those they study pose one of the greatest threats to these methodological strengths. Such inequalities have an extensive history in anthropology, and by the 1970s and especially the 1980s, many anthropologists were engaging in considerable self-reflection about the power politics involved in ethnographic knowledge production (e.g., Asad 1995; Marcus and Fischer 1986). Native American activists had visibly raised these issues even earlier, however. Vine Deloria Jr.'s famous essay "Anthropologists and Other Friends," originally printed in *Custer Died for Your Sins* in 1969 (Deloria 1988), was perhaps the most widely disseminated call for greater accountability to Native communities by anthropologists. Ethnographic work in Native

North America was virtually a rite of passage for many professional anthropologists educated in the United States before the 1960s, but following these calls such work became far less popular. I was advised more than once as a graduate student in the early 1990s to consider working elsewhere, for example, given the hostility and difficulty that many professors felt I was sure to encounter as a non-Native researcher.

Calls for local relevance move to redress a long-standing imbalance of power within ethnographic research in Native North America, however, and it seems likely that they will eventually characterize ethnographic work in most, if not all, settings. Moreover, I soon found that while hostility was a recurrent feature of my experience at Northern Cheyenne, it was by no means pervasive. I simply tried to avoid selected community members who were well known for their insulting and antagonizing demeanor toward non-Natives. I did not always succeed, ending up in the line of fire of one such person when I helped with a community sobriety campout and received some positive public acknowledgment from event organizers at one point. Such instances were isolated and relatively easy for me to categorize as such, however. For the most part, I overwhelmingly experienced social grace, good humor, and the ability to share a laugh with Northern Cheyenne community members. I also experienced a wide range of responses to the fact that I was a health researcher and specifically an anthropologist, from support to suspicion to disinterest.

My efforts to interact with knowledgeable or politically significant local actors in some aspect of what I was studying sometimes met, for example, with highly scripted comments that reflected locally conventionalized modes of interacting with people in whatever ethnic, gender, and/or age categories were salient in their perceptions of me. The ways in which age and gender orient social interactions on the reservation made it difficult for me to spend enough time around some categories of people to build the rapport necessary to move beyond such conventionalized interactions.

In ethnographic fieldwork even such conventionalized encounters can serve as important sources of information, however. For example, others' positioning of me in their social world helped me to learn more about local attitudes toward sexuality and sexual diversity, and perceptions of non-Natives. In my twenties and unmarried at the time of my initial work in the 1990s, my long-distance relationship at the time clearly did not impress most Cheyennes that I knew, and ended up being a source of considerable commentary and teasing, as women would encourage me to get married, and some younger men would ask me how come I would not go out with them if I was not wearing a ring. On one occasion shortly after my arrival, from what I gleaned from the conversation in Cheyenne, an older man who ran a health program for which I was volunteering jokingly offered to exchange me in marriage to an elderly male client, as an incentive for improving his diabetes control!

One of the closest friendships that I formed on the reservation was with a woman who was rumored to have a history of same-sex romantic relationships. As years passed and my long-distance relationship eventually did founder, I was rather surprised to learn that many people on the reservation assumed that I must be engaged in a sexual relationship with her. My own socially liberal upbringing, as well as a long-standing, close friendship with a man who is gay, had led me to treat sexual orientation as a feature of a person's life that did not have much bearing on whether or not we shared enough common ground to be friends. My training in ethnographic methods did not provide much in the way of skills to respond to the cultural divide between my own attitudes here, however, and those of Northern Cheyenne community members who seemed quite convinced of their own perceptions. While I was in the field, Lewin and Leap's *Out in the Field: Reflections of Lesbian and Gay Anthropologists* (1996) was published to address the unique situations that sexual-minority ethnographers can encounter during fieldwork. Looking through it, I was bemused by how these needed conversations within the discipline still did not equip those of us experiencing the social awkwardness of an erroneous "outing" to respond effectively! So long as this particular friendship continued, it seemed, these local perceptions of me would also.

However socially awkward they may be, such misperceptions can be ethnographically informative. Local cultural assumptions about the nature and importance of sexuality were evident in how long-distance relationships and lengthy periods of celibacy, while not terribly unusual in the lives of academics that I know, were clearly not recognized as realistic possibilities for organizing one's romantic life from the perspectives of some Northern Cheyennes. Assumptions also seem evident here that non-Natives who stay in the community for extended periods of time must be deriving some clear and immediate personal gratification from their presence. A Northern Cheyenne health administrator once spontaneously commented to me that from his perspective, most non-Natives who came and stayed for lengthy periods of time in the community were "running from something." (With characteristic local humor, another participant in the conversation then immediately quipped, "We just hope it's not the law!") The administrator's turn of phrase interestingly puts the primary emphasis on what is being avoided ("running from"), positioning what the community is and what it offers as only secondary in the motivations of the non-Natives in question.

My own minor experience of being misinterpreted also served as an entry point to a better understanding of attitudes and interpretations that hold far greater significance in the lives of reservation community members. In a departure from the attitudes of tolerance toward sexual diversity that is documented in early ethnographies about the Cheyennes (e.g., Grinnell 1972a [1923]), attitudes on the reservation by the 1990s included tendencies to stigmatize nonheterosexual relationships, marking them as topics for negative gossip. Indeed, through the course of fieldwork I found that many Cheyennes who are not or not exclusively heterosexual in their relationships tend to avoid talking about these issues openly. Some who openly live with same-sex partners experience harassment, an element of the broader political dynamics of reservation life that I discuss further in the chapters that follow.

Since I anticipated considerable local ambivalence about my social identity as a non-Native researcher, I invested considerable time and energy in establishing rapport, making myself visible around the community by volunteering with a community health outreach worker program and teaching social science courses at the tribal community college. I also engaged in participant observation at Recovery Center (the reservation's central substance abuse service program), at various recovery-related community events and Twelve Step meetings, and in a variety of other family and community settings.

I conducted my first formal semistructured interviews as part of a small project of 20 interviews with staff and clients at Recovery Center, which included both men and women. I subsequently expanded to include a broader community-based sample of women, completing more unstructured life history interviews with a total of 35 women who self-identified as either being sober or pursuing sobriety. The women ranged in age from 18 to 84, with the majority in their forties and fifties.

Both in the mid-1990s and during a follow-up study in 2005, I then conducted semistructured interviews with 23 staff members in reservation health care programs. These emphasized questions about the complexities of local self-determination in health services and drew from my experience as a volunteer with the Community Health Representatives (a paraprofessional community health outreach program) from 1994 to 1996 and as an employee within Community Health Programs from 1996 to 1997 (working primarily with the Tribal Nutrition program, but also conducting data analysis for other programs and projects). I attended or helped to plan numerous health-related trainings, workshops, and community events on the reservation throughout this era. Many of the lasting friendships that I have developed on the reservation also involve health care staff, and we have continued to stay in touch over the years by phone and e-mail, as well as when I return to Montana or when they visit me while traveling to workshops or visiting relatives off the reservation. I selected interviewees here in part based on these ongoing social connections but also solicited input from people that I did not know well personally but knew would help to represent the broad range of local perspectives about the challenges of providing health care on the reservation.

Central Questions

Three central questions orient this book. First, how do efforts to define and address alcohol-related problems at Northern Cheyenne take shape in a distinctive local cultural landscape? Part I includes two chapters that consider how a distinctive historical consciousness informs local perceptions of threats to collective well-being, outlines the key rhetorical frameworks involved, and examines how these are visible in the range of local responses to alcohol—including critical commentary about Twelve Step approaches to sobriety. These discussions highlight the multiple and contested meanings of sobriety on the reservation, and how responses to alcohol are embedded within broader political processes in local community life.

The three chapters in part II examine two additional major questions: How and why are Twelve Step approaches alienating to many community members, but creatively and selectively adapted by some—most notably, women of younger generations? Moreover, how and why do institutionalized services to support sobriety on the reservation remain oriented around the Twelve Steps, despite clear evidence of grassroots efforts toward alternatives and widespread local recognition of the need for more culturally appropriate approaches? These chapters are centered on a detailed analysis of psychocultural themes in women's narratives about their lives, coupled with ethnographic observations of community responses to the grassroots efforts to modify Twelve Step approaches that some younger-generation women are undertaking. Examining sobriety in these ways speaks to broader anthropological questions of how social and political processes intersect with subjective experience and its expression.

A final ethnographic chapter and short conclusion in part III then revisit the implications of this analysis for providing culturally appropriate services for alcohol-related health problems within Native North American communities like Northern Cheyenne. In theory, local control and culturally relevant adaptations of such services are now possible throughout Native North America. Accounts by Northern Cheyenne health staff and community leaders portray serious practical barriers to achieving both, however. Their perspectives speak to ongoing concerns in medical anthropology about how power relations shape the production of knowledge about health and demonstrate how ethnographic studies of drinking and sobriety in Native North America can benefit from closer attention to these issues.

Part I
Understanding Alcohol in Cultural Context

While critiques of Twelve Step approaches to sobriety are certainly not unique to Northern Cheyenne, they are nonetheless situated within a distinctive cultural context on the reservation. Local consciousness of past collective experiences, and rhetorical tools for comparing past with present, animate community conversations about alcohol and other contemporary social problems in ways that are locally distinctive.

To understand the local meanings of historical references and the significance of how they are made first requires a critical awareness of prominent American cultural narratives of "how the West was won." Many students, friends, and academic colleagues that I encounter seem unaware of the extent to which communities like Northern Cheyenne continue to experience persistent inequalities relative to non-Natives in the United States and consequently either view Native Americans who make historical references as inexplicably "living in the past" or express confusion about why past experiences remain important in a post–Civil Rights era of purportedly equal opportunity. In turn, those who are aware of the breadth of ongoing inequalities in Native North America often express a sense of resignation, as if these are so entrenched as to be inevitable. Such responses say more about the ongoing power of Euro-American colonial ideologies in U.S. cultural life, and an associated persistent ambivalence about the rights and special legal status of Native Americans, than they do about the historical experiences of North American tribes and historical consciousness in contemporary Native communities.

While the specific imagery of heathen brutes, Noble Savages, and so forth in U.S. cultural narratives of Native American experiences has shifted over time, a continuing reliance on stereotyped historical portraits has consistently worked to limit available information about the contemporary realities of Native peoples. Pearce argues that in Euro-American narratives throughout the nineteenth century, Native Americans were effectively "forced out of American life into American history" (1988:58), and Berkhofer documents how twentieth-century American cultural narratives continued to produce "ahistorical and static" (1978:29) constructions of "Indians" as antithetical to esteemed cultural notions of adaptation and progress.

These assumptions orient popular responses to the historical references made by indigenous peoples themselves, which circulate in numerous public arenas from media outlets to courts and claims commissions to scholarship. Efforts to integrate or sometimes privilege Native North American perspectives on their historical experiences have become widespread, visible not only in efforts by Native activists pursuing political and legal claims (e.g., Johnson 2008:97), but also in a wealth of scholarship in Native American studies (Edmunds 1995; Fixico 1997; Mihesuah and Wilson 2004; Shoemaker 2002). In both my professional and personal lives, I continually encounter non-Natives who assume that Native Americans are either fully passive victims or empowered actors, rather than appreciating the subtle continuum in between. Yet the complexities of indigenous experiences often do not fit either characterization. To emplot indigenous experience on either course reflects broader cultural efforts to frame Euro-American colonialism as somehow inevitable, if tragic, or to deny that its legacies persist. The political and moral work accomplished by such historical accounts warrants critical scrutiny.

When topics turn to alcohol use by Native North Americans, universalizing explanations that overlook localized histories of when and how drinking became widespread are very common. So too are interpretations that overlook or misinterpret the politics of competing perspectives on alcohol within a reservation community such as Northern Cheyenne. These broad generalizations and their underlying moral assumptions about Native experiences and health also deserve close attention.

To examine these issues, the following two chapters move between my own ethnographic material and published historical and ethnohistorical accounts to argue that a distinctive historical consciousness has emerged at Northern Cheyenne from collective experiences of colonization, followed by persistent economic, political, and cultural marginalization within the social order of the United States. Prominent local rhetorical conventions for characterizing threats to Cheyenne well-being have emerged through experiences of collective dispossession and have set parameters for localized debates about the specific problem of alcohol. Indeed, the fact that a prominent term for alcohol in the Cheyenne language translates as "white man's water" attests to local perceptions of the close relationship between colonization and alcohol use.

Recent social theory has called for greater attention to ambiguity and complexity in power relations under colonialism, appreciating the diversity of local histories due to the reciprocal influence between colonizer and colonized (e.g., Cohn 1996; Comaroff and Comaroff 2003). At the same time, study of colonialism and its aftermath includes appreciating the perpetuation of profound structural inequalities alongside the persistence of cultural distinctiveness among indigenous peoples. While a full historical analysis of these interactions at Northern Cheyenne is beyond the scope of this book, the following chapters help to emphasize the importance of historical legacies for contemporary reservation life and for the political dynamics of community responses to alcohol.

Chapter 2 describes prominent local rhetorical conventions for characterizing threats to well-being, and how these reflect a distinctive historical consciousness that is grounded in legacies of experiencing and often resisting dispossession. It also outlines the increasing diversity of social experiences within the Northern Cheyenne community as a key historical process that has sparked ambivalent responses from reservation community members The multiple moral worlds that result produce competing claims about history and identity that in turn infuse local debates about how to define and address social problems. Different types of monolithic claims about "Cheyenne culture" that overlook or pathologize diversity have multiple origins, motivations, and effects, but they have all been shaped by the discursive and material pressures that originated with early colonial administrative agencies. These have been perpetuated through subsequent federal policy shifts through the present era of self-determination and tend either to obscure the current diversity and complexity of the community or to construct it as evidence of pathology.

While it takes different forms and has diverse effects, one consequence of misrecognizing the pluralism in local moral worlds on the reservation in institutionalized health services has been to undermine their cultural relevance. Chapter 3 looks specifically at how these rhetorical conventions and associated politics are visible in local interpretations of and responses to alcohol, and introduces how alcohol services based on the Twelve Steps of Alcoholics Anonymous face special challenges here in large part because they do not accommodate the local realities of social and psychological diversity among community members.

Key Resources: Northern Cheyenne Experiences

Material within the following chapters variously affirms, extends, and debates findings from a variety of published works about the Northern Cheyennes. Under the auspices of 1970s state legislation to improve public education about the history of Montana's Native peoples, historian Tom Weist worked closely with Northern Cheyenne leadership in the 1970s to produce a new ethnohistorical account (1977) that explicitly aimed to represent local perspectives that were overlooked in previous historical and anthropological scholarship. Weist also worked to publish historical observations made by attentive and sympathetic non-Natives in the community, such as Thomas Marquis (Marquis 1978), who initially came to the reservation as an agency physician in the early decades of the twentieth century but ended up producing a wealth of ethnographic and ethnohistorical texts and photographs.

Local anthropologist Margot Liberty has produced several richly descriptive ethnohistorical works about the Northern Cheyennes. These include a collaborative book (1998) with tribal historian John Stands in Timber (1882–1967) and, most recently (Marquis et al. 2007), a book based on Marquis's early-twentieth-century photographs at Northern Cheyenne, with interpretations that Liberty developed collaboratively with the influential Northern Cheyenne leader John Woodenlegs (1910–81).

A variety of other scholars have written ethnographies and ethnohistories of the Cheyennes, all working within the major theoretical paradigms of their times. Naturalist George Bird Grinnell produced several meticulously detailed volumes in the late-nineteenth-/early-twentieth-century vein of "salvage anthropology," based on interviews and observations in the early reservation years (1972a, 1972b). Anthropologist E. Adamson Hoebel produced numerous ethnographic studies of the Cheyennes through the middle twentieth century, including an interesting study of jurisprudence coauthored with Karl Llewellyn (1941), and a much more well-known ethnographic case study of the Cheyennes (1978) that reflects the culture and personality approach of early American anthropology. Despite its resulting limitations, this case study has remained one of the most widely read ethnographic accounts of the tribe.

Peter J. Powell, a Jesuit priest and scholar, conducted fieldwork primarily among the Northern Cheyennes from the 1950s to the 1970s and has produced two extensive two-volume sets about Cheyenne religious beliefs and practices (1969, 1981). While generally constructing an argument about the parallels between Cheyenne views and Christianity, these texts are centered on observations and interviews with Cheyenne men with extensive knowledge of ceremonial lore and offer a wealth of descriptive information about ritual practices and associated community debates.

Anthropologist John Moore, working from a political-economic perspective and primarily among the Southern Cheyennes from the late 1970s, has produced a detailed history of Cheyenne social and political organization (1987), as well as a shorter overview of past and present lifeways (1999). Katherine (Toby) Weist conducted her doctoral dissertation fieldwork at Northern Cheyenne in the late 1960s and produced a detailed life history narrative of tribal member Belle Highwalking (1982) that was also published through the Montana state initiative described above. Anne (Terry) Straus also conducted ethnographic fieldwork on the Northern Cheyenne Reservation, with an emphasis in symbolic anthropology (1976) and a strong ethnopsychological focus (1977).

Since the 1980s sociologist Carol Ward and colleagues have conducted a mixture of quantitative and qualitative research while working closely with the local tribal college, Chief Dull Knife College, and the Tribal Education Program. Although Ward's major work (2005) concerns schooling and human capital in relation to economic development, she completed a qualitative project about women and sobriety that overlapped my own in the 1990s (Baird-Olson and Ward 2000), after recognizing how this trend was impacting Northern Cheyenne women's educational participation.

Finally, I also draw briefly on personal accounts of experiences on the Northern Cheyenne Reservation produced by Stella (Sunny) Peters (1992) and Jerry Mader (2002). Peters produced a locally published book of recollections based on her decades of work as a nurse on the reservation starting in the 1940s. Photographer Mader worked with Tom Weist on local history projects in the 1970s and later published a memoir through a university press, the proceeds of which support historical preservation projects through Chief Dull Knife College.

2
Misrecognizing Local Moral Worlds

Daily conversation on the Northern Cheyenne Reservation features numerous themes of both experiencing and witnessing a variety of troubling social problems. Limited economic resources; domestic conflicts; community violence; capriciousness in local governance, justice, and service systems; and efforts to cope with disease, disability, and premature death are among the most common topics. While these discussions often mention drinking, some people implicate alcohol as a primary cause of these problems, while others treat it as merely a component. Discussions of alcohol at Northern Cheyenne are therefore situated within wider-ranging critical commentary about reservation life, much of which links current community problems with the tribe's collective historical experience of colonization. Examining the rhetorical features and social consequences of how such historical references are made demonstrates how a distinctive historical consciousness, or "culturally patterned way or ways of experiencing and understanding history" (Ohnuki-Tierney 1990:4), infuses social life on the Northern Cheyenne Reservation and shapes the stories that many community members tell about contemporary problems.

Historical references are commonly made both at public events and in daily conversation and tend to explicitly compare and contrast past Cheyenne lifeways with present experiences. Ethnographers working in a variety of postcolonial contexts have noted local tendencies to draw contrasts between an "idealized past and discordant present" (Comaroff and Comaroff 1987:193), and thereby link current experiences of inequality and marginalization with past injustices. In drawing such historical contrasts, speakers articulate not only critiques of colonialism but also their moral worlds, or the subjective senses of what is good, right, desirable, and expected that shapes how they interpret the flow of their daily experiences. O'Nell (1996) describes, for example, how stories of historical events told by Flathead (Salish-Kootenai) Reservation community members in western Montana reinforce key themes in their accounts of current interactions with non-Natives, to remind all present how the sociopolitical dominance of non-Natives in Flathead lands and lives continues to threaten the survival of key local moral values of endurance, humor, generosity, kinship ties, and respect for the natural world. At Northern Cheyenne historical references similarly invest images of past lifeways with high value and emphasize how key local moral values from the past remain essential under the often troubling conditions of contemporary life.

As statements that assert a morally vested vision of what community members should be doing, thinking, or feeling in their daily lives and experiences, however, historical references often provoke intense debate at Northern Cheyenne. Such conflicts highlight how the community is constituted by multiple moral worlds rather than a singular cultural world of shared values, beliefs, and practices. Controversies arise due, in part, to numerous social and psychological differences among community members, but also because much of the flow of local social interaction on the reservation is explicitly politicized by a constant need to define and defend local rights. As in numerous other Native North American (Champagne 2007) and indigenous communities worldwide (Cultural Survival 2007), many Northern Cheyenne community members devote considerable time and energy to preserving lands, enhancing political autonomy, and maintaining cultural distinctiveness from the surrounding non-Native society in the face of powerful and recurrent pressures to the contrary. References that contrast past Cheyenne lifeways with present conditions imbue change, loss, and community responses to both with layers of moral meaning that can inspire action as well as spark debate.

When historical references provoke controversy at Northern Cheyenne, critics usually do not explicitly take issue with the values articulated in stories about the past. Instead, they most often challenge the accuracy of the story, how the speaker relates it to contemporary issues, and/or whether the speaker really has the social authority that is locally required to make claims about how things are or should be. O'Nell's study on the Flathead Reservation also elegantly describes how debates linking social authority to cultural identity permeate daily life and feature a key local discursive convention that she defines as "the rhetoric of the empty center" (1996:55). Using a heuristic diagram of concentric circles to illustrate, O'Nell explains how the empty circle at the center marks the passing of the "real Indians" of an idealized precolonial past, and the concentric rings indicate how community members' claims variably position themselves and others as closer to or farther away from this moral center. A similar rhetoric is widely evident at Northern Cheyenne, but here prophecies by the culture hero Sweet Medicine also serve as a key rhetorical device. These prophecies explicitly pose thorny questions about whether and how it is possible to remain Cheyenne under the pressures imposed by American colonization, lending a special intensity to the comparison between past and present that in turn infuses how claims link cultural identity and social authority at Northern Cheyenne.

Anthropological approaches to history often focus on how multiple and competing tellings of past events or processes emerge as people "respond to the conflicting exigencies of their social, political, and cultural predicaments" (Herzfeld 2001:55). At Northern Cheyenne, as in many other indigenous communities, people must contend with the central predicament of how the imposition of non-Native interpretations of indigenous experiences, through everything from reservation administration to popular media, has shaped the evolving course of local cultural modes of interpreting experience.

Historical Consciousness in Action

Tribal history is commemorated through organized tribal holidays and community-based events at Northern Cheyenne, as well as in the flow of everyday social life. The local significance of the past is embodied in the institutionalization of an office devoted to historical preservation in the administrative structure of the Northern Cheyenne Tribe. Its staff members largely deal with the cultural resource management components of environmental and archaeological projects that relate to tribal history but have also monitored how Cheyenne experiences are represented in museums and have contributed to several recent efforts to designate key nineteenth-century sites as national historic monuments (see below). Other local institutions on or near the reservation have also developed Northern Cheyenne heritage centers, museums, and oral history projects, ranging from the tribal community college[1] to a long-standing local Catholic school (St. Labre Indian School). As a result, the local community features multiple and often different public representations of Cheyenne history.

These local public histories share an emphasis on commemorating nineteenth-century events and experiences. Yet interestingly, despite this institutional emphasis, no detailed and accessible narrative history of this century seems to have circulated within the community at large since the reservation was established. Detailed public knowledge about nineteenth-century military successes against the Americans is especially limited.[2] Experiences of dislocation and trauma may well have constrained whether and how such stories were passed on, and U.S. federal policies of prosecution for war crimes in the early reservation years clearly also contributed. Instead, select individuals have been locally recognized as having specialized knowledge about tribal history. Joe Walksalong (ca. 1930–2004), well known locally as the first Northern Cheyenne to become a minister in the Mennonite church, was asked to offer a series of evening lectures about Cheyenne historical experiences and social traditions at the tribal college in the mid-1990s. Others have been appointed to more formal roles as tribal historians, such as John Stands in Timber (1882–1967) and Bill Tallbull (1921–96). In the 1990s Tallbull taught oral history and ethnobotany classes at the tribal college, served as a consultant on projects related to regional historic sites relevant to the Cheyennes, and was active in other cultural and environmental preservation efforts.

The emphasis on nineteenth-century Cheyenne lifeways and experiences in these roles and activities bears at least superficial similarities to broader North American popular interest in how Native peoples figured within the story of "how the West was won" in the mid- to late 1800s on the Great Plains. Several classic ethnographies and histories of the Cheyennes have circulated widely as part of this fascination with "Plains Indians," and generations of U.S. undergraduates have encountered Hoebel's 1978 anthropological case study *The Cheyennes: Indians of the Great Plains,* especially.

A cursory reading of any of these texts yields a portrait of how nineteenth-century Cheyenne men hunted buffalo and earned social prestige through raiding for horses and defending hunting territories and other resources from enemy tribes. Women processed the products of the hunt into food, domestic articles, and trade goods; gathered vegetables and fruits; and reared children with assistance from female kin. Men were the major players in a system of governance that was relatively unique on the Plains, involving a centralized Council of Forty-four Chiefs in addition to the soldier or military societies that were widespread across

Plains tribes. The Council of Forty-four Chiefs made decisions affecting the whole tribe, and its membership consisted largely of band leaders.

Bands were extended family groups that lived semiautonomously for much of the year but gathered together once each summer in a massive camp circle for a collective buffalo hunt, the performance of major collective religious ceremonies, and meetings of the Council of Forty-four Chiefs. The men's military societies were sodalities whose memberships cut across the different bands and dealt with decisions and activities relating to war and with the strategic use of violence within the tribe (e.g., policing the collective buffalo hunts).

These economic practices and social institutions were linked with a broader cosmology that hinged upon a notion of energy or power that emerged from the Creator, Ma?heo?o, and coursed through various levels in a hierarchy of spiritual beings (Moore 1999; Powell 1969). Human beings could access this power at various levels of the hierarchy through sacrificial acts such as fasting and piercing,[3] which were often vowed by a person facing hard times (e.g., Grinnell 1972a:79–85, Stands in Timber and Liberty 1998:93). Two culture heroes brought two sacred objects and associated rituals and teachings to the Cheyennes. Sweet Medicine received instruction from spiritual powers at a site in the Black Hills region about the ethics and practices necessary for success in a lifeway of hunting and raiding. In passing along these teachings, he gave the people four stone-tipped Sacred Arrows. Erect Horns brought the Sacred Buffalo Hat, which houses a female buffalo spirit. These sacred objects each required constant attendance by a specially appointed Keeper. The proper ritual care of the Sacred Arrows was implicated in the success of nineteenth-century hunting and war parties, while tending appropriately to the Sacred Buffalo Hat ensured the reproduction of the Cheyennes, the animals upon which they depended, and the broader cosmos of which all were a part.

Most classic works about the Cheyennes also emphasize their well-known armed resistance to American colonization (e.g., Grinnell 1956). Moore notes how U.S. soldiers faced Cheyenne warriors in nearly half (nine out of twenty-one) of the battles involving the highest U.S. casualties in the "Indian Wars" of the American West between 1837 and 1891 (1999:103). These include the 1876 Battle of the Little Bighorn, site of George Armstrong Custer's famous strategic error when confronting a massive assembly of Lakota, Cheyenne, and Arapaho warriors.

All major ethnographies about the Cheyennes also describe how a division of the tribe into Northern and Southern groups emerged in the early nineteenth century. Initiated as some bands pursued horse and buffalo herds far to the south, this division intensified as American colonial activity interfered with both buffalo migrations and Native freedom of travel up and down the plains, and was formally recognized by tribal members in the 1840s (Hoebel 1978:10). As Moore (1999) describes, by the mid-nineteenth century a course of treaty making and peace tended to be emphasized by Southern Cheyennes, a pattern of raiding by a Cheyenne military society called the Dog Soldiers, and the armed defense of a hunting lifeway by the Northern Cheyennes; and personal preferences as well as major events could inspire people to shift their identities and allegiances among the three.

The northern bands of the Cheyennes did not surrender to U.S. forces until 1877. They were then led to the Oklahoma reservation of the southern bands under armed guard, where they remained from May to September 1878. Two groups, led by chiefs Morning Star (better known by his teasing nickname, Dull Knife) and Little Wolf, then embarked on an epic flight back north. Diplomacy by Two Moons and other Northern Cheyennes already working as U.S. Army scouts in the north, coupled with supportive advocacy by Colonel Miles from Fort Keogh (see Stands in Timber and Liberty 1998:239), ultimately succeeded in procuring an Executive Order from President Chester A. Arthur to establish the Tongue River Reservation in southeastern Montana in November of 1884, later renamed the Northern Cheyenne Reservation. By the early 1890s, various groups of Northern Cheyennes had settled, roughly along band lines, in regions that soon became identified as "districts" of the reservation.[4]

While basically accurate, this cursory portrait is also highly selective, conveying an image of cultural coherence in nineteenth-century Cheyenne life that is complicated by closer readings of both classic and less widely known works about this era of Cheyenne history (see below). The primary cultural significance of collective history lies in how past events and experiences are referenced and reconstructed in response to current concerns (see also Comaroff and Comaroff 1992; Hobsbawm and Ranger 1983)—and the localized politics that result.

Contested Histories

While the goals of Northern Cheyenne commemorative activities vary, many share in the broader agenda of promoting alternatives to the prevalent representations of nineteenth-century U.S. history that tribal

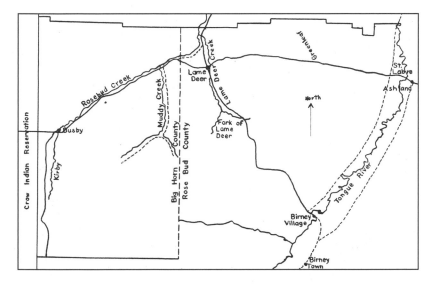

Figure 3. Map of the Northern Cheyenne Reservation. The tribe maintains a policy of prohibition on reservation lands, but off-reservation bars are located within a quarter mile of the northern and eastern borders and within a mile of the southern border. Reprinted with permission from Weist, 1977.

members have encountered in textbooks, Hollywood movies, and museums, as well as in myriad social interactions with non-Natives. Younger generations of Northern Cheyennes especially emphasize the power of these images in their early lives. One young man told me how he played "cowboys and Indians" in his front yard while growing up in the reservation village of Busby and now laughed at the irony of how he always wanted to play the character that he felt was the hero: Custer! Several women described going as children to powwows and other community events that involved dancing and drumming, and impatiently complaining while waiting for things to start, "I want to see the Indians!" With amusement they recalled how their annoyed mothers responded, "Hush now, we *are* Indian!" These stories describe the complexities of coming to terms with one's Cheyenne identity, in the face of numerous encounters with negative and/or stereotyped images of "Indians."

In addition to undermining the force of popular stereotypes in tribal members' experiences and self-concepts, historical references play key roles in efforts to raise broader public awareness about past injustices experienced by the Cheyennes. Recent successful activism by Northern Cheyenne community members, for example, helped to establish a national historic monument at the site of an 1864 massacre of Cheyennes encamped at Sand Creek in southeastern Colorado (U.S. Department of the Interior, National Park Service 2009). The ways in which their efforts quickly sparked debates with local non-Natives also illustrate the political stakes that continue to surround representations of U.S. history.

By nearly all accounts, the 1864 camp of Cheyennes at Sand Creek was a peaceful one, and its leader, Black Kettle, had raised both a white flag and a U.S. flag to communicate this status. Yet American forces in this era sometimes used profoundly racialized logics to rationalize attacking any Cheyennes that they could find in retaliation for acts that they knew or thought had been committed by others. Colorado state militia forces unleashed a devastating early morning assault on the camp.

Beginning in the 1990s a group of Northern Cheyenne descendants of those present at this massacre advocated, in collaboration with the Southern Cheyennes and Arapahoes and with officials of the Northern Cheyenne Tribe, to gain recognition of Sand Creek as a national historic site. The organizers describe their goals as honoring the experiences of their ancestors through memorial, and promoting awareness of the injustice of the violence that occurred at this site. Controversies soon arose between the activists and local non-Natives at the site, however, including debates over whether it was more accurate to follow the Cheyennes in calling the event a massacre or to use the less evocative term *battle*. After more than a decade of negotiations, the site opened to the public in spring 2007. I was able to visit a couple of months later and noticed that the various participants agreed to disagree in that the site's name uses the term "massacre," but some of the informational markers use "battle" and present competing views of the event. While the non-Natives' desire to defend the honor of their ancestors is perhaps understandable, their stake in the public representation of events at Sand Creek may reflect broader U.S. cultural tensions. The vocal claims of civil rights activism both nationally and internationally have raised popular awareness of claims that link past injustice with contemporary social inequalities. These claims contradict key U.S. cultural concepts of meritocracy ("everyone gets to the station in life that they earn"), individualism ("pull yourself up by your own bootstraps"), and progress ("discrimination used to be a problem, but it isn't anymore"). Even the implication that past injustices may have legacies for the present can therefore inspire responses ranging from concern to skepticism to hostility among adherents to these ideologies. For Northern Cheyenne activists, such responses perpetuate troubling public ignorance and/or disinterest regarding the political and economic marginalization that, to them, was initiated in early colonial experiences and has been perpetuated ever since.

Indeed, critical commentary on the reservation routinely targets local conditions ranging from the less-than-palatable government commodity foods that are familiar to every reservation resident, to the fast-deteriorating and sometimes oddly colored government surplus paint used in reservation housing. Stories of erratic decisions and mismanagement by federal agencies or their staff members are common, as are claims about the poor quality of some teachers, health care staff, and other non-Natives who come to work on the reservation. Whether or not such attributions are accurate in particular cases, they suggest that continual experiences of disenfranchisement form a significant psychological reality for many community members. Such stories are variously told with humor that highlights the absurdities at hand or with bitterness that emphasizes the very real human suffering that reservation conditions can produce (see also Mader 2002; Moore 1999; O'Nell 1996).

Themes of invisibility and marginalization are especially intense when Northern Cheyenne community members talk about their experiences in the health care system. Frustration with long waiting times, limited funds, and brusque interactions with some non-Native clinical staff are common themes in commentary about local services. Cheyenne friends also recount discriminatory practices in health care settings off the reservation. In one case, a family that had recently endured the trauma of losing a baby to medical error by hospital staff at a regional medical center soon found themselves in another off-reservation hospital after several relatives were seriously injured in a car accident. Adults in the family sent a highly intelligent child of about eight years old to get information from the nursing staff, who promptly assumed that the child was lost and unsupervised and called in the hospital social worker to reprimand the family. Hospital staff failed to recognize the culturally distinctive styles of family organization and patterns of entrusting individuals with responsibility at work here, and instead operated from stereotyped assumptions about neglectful Native parenting. Their resulting actions compounded the extreme levels of stress already being experienced by the family.

Much of this critical commentary by Northern Cheyennes highlights the limited control that community members have over the perceptions and actions of non-Natives, as well as over the political and economic forces that shape local conditions on the reservation. Politically, the chiefs council and military societies continue to influence reservation governance; their actions and sources of authority are less institutionalized than those of the elected tribal government. The latter was formed in the 1930s and is modeled on the U.S. political system, and its decision making continues to be overseen by the federal Bureau of Indian Affairs. Moreover, much of the local economy has remained dependent upon federal funding since the reservation was established. The Northern Cheyennes were not offered any workable replacement for their lost hunting livelihood in the early reservation years but instead received inadequate food rations and pressures to engage in small-scale farming that was poorly suited to the dry climate and short growing seasons of the northern Plains. They were also subjected to federal mismanagement that undermined irrigation projects and a successful tribal cattle enterprise (see Weist 1977). The general economic decline in the rural United States over the twentieth century further limited economic opportunities on the reservation. All of these factors coalesced such that by the end of the twentieth century, federally funded education, health, and social service programs continued to generate the overwhelming majority of available jobs on the reservation (e.g., Ward and Wilson 1989). A variety of tribal programs have worked to generate and sustain small businesses on the reservation, and tribal leaders helped to successfully acquire the first bank on reservation land in the late 1990s to help support these enterprises and diversify the local economy. Unemployment and underemployment have remained common, however, with tribal agency reports in the 1990s documenting seasonal unemployment rates as high as 68 percent.[5]

With this combination of political and economic factors, living on the Northern Cheyenne Reservation involves constant encounters with the vagaries of federal policy. Transitions between presidential administrations are often accompanied by changes in federal policy and/or in the levels of funding for existing policies, for instance, which translates locally into concrete events such as losses or gains in health programs, social services, and employment for reservation residents.

To characterize reservation conditions as life on the margins is not to say that efforts by Northern Cheyennes to defend rights and resources are never effective, however. Local activism in the 1970s successfully asserted local priorities and values to cancel plans for large-scale coal mining. As Champagne (1989) describes, the Northern Cheyennes were among many tribes whose lands were targeted for potential fossil fuel development during the international energy crisis of the 1970s. Community-based opponents of the Bureau of Indian Affairs' plans to mine the coal argued that the large scale of the proposed extraction would profoundly change not only the physical but also the cultural landscape of the reservation. They lent rhetorical force to their case by emphasizing how the land was sacred, symbolic of the cultural integrity and survival of the tribe, and hard-won by Northern Cheyenne ancestors. The mining leases that had been signed were canceled, and the tribe approved more limited plans to drill for natural gas that brought money and employment without anywhere near the environmental damage of the proposed mining plans.

Other key Northern Cheyenne successes in asserting local priorities have included land claims and defenses against non-Native appropriations of Cheyenne spiritual beliefs and ritual practices. Key tribal leader John Woodenlegs negotiated a major land purchase when reservation lands that had been sold to non-Cheyennes came up for sale in the late 1950s, and he was instrumental in a successful major Indian Claims Commission case in the early 1960s to redress land losses due to treaty violations (Weist 1977). The 1972 publication of Hyemeyohsts Storm's book *Seven Arrows,* which claimed to represent fundamental Cheyenne spiritual beliefs and practices, provoked Northern and Southern Cheyenne leaders to file a complaint with its publisher over numerous inaccuracies in the text. In response, Harper and Row edited out the offending passages in later editions and paid a cash settlement (see Mader 2002). Activism against New Age appropriations of Native spirituality continued through the efforts of Austin Two Moons and other Northern Cheyennes in the 1980s, who published a statement on how to distinguish a legitimate Native American ritual practitioner from a "plastic medicine man" (Churchill 1992).

Yet at Northern Cheyenne such successes are counterbalanced by an ongoing stream of experiences in which local perspectives and priorities are overlooked or disregarded. Community members have worked with mixed success to protect sites sacred to their own and other tribes on the northern Plains. Native rights to such sites were sometimes recognized in local treaties and are rhetorically affirmed by the American Indian Religious Freedom Act of 1978 (amended in 1993) but in practice often

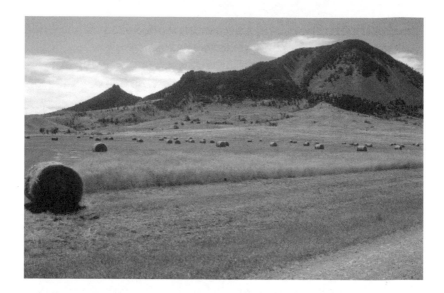

Figure 4. Bear Butte (Noahå-vose). Photo by the author.

conflict with the economic and recreational priorities of non-Natives. Bear Butte in the Black Hills region of South Dakota is the site where the key Cheyenne culture hero Sweet Medicine received instruction from spiritual powers. Around World War II Northern Cheyennes began going there to conduct rituals of fasting (Powell 1981), many of which take place in the summer months. Dates in early August overlap, however, with the massive annual motorcycle rally at nearby Sturgis, South Dakota.

While Northern Cheyennes that I accompanied to Bear Butte during the Sturgis rally were often extremely amused by the glaring conflict between their spiritual aims and the sex/drugs/rock-and-roll focus of the bikers, they were also troubled when noise and light from the festivities disrupted the contemplation and listening required during fasting. In 2005 a local saloon owner proposed building a new bar that would be closer to the butte than any previous establishment. While the butte itself is protected as a state park and national historic landmark, the lands surrounding it are owned by local ranchers and have been open to development. Northern Cheyennes participated in protests and petitioning to block this new enterprise. The new bar was ultimately built, however, and was visibly open for business during the rally when I last visited Bear Butte in summer of 2008.

Ongoing experiences such as these communicate to all Northern Cheyennes that respect for their priorities and perspectives is by no means guaranteed. Yet community members frequently disagree about how to respond. More detailed examples of how historical references can generate debate and controversy on the reservation illustrate this local diversity.

Commemorative Practices and Local Controversies

By the 1990s several nineteenth-century events had come to figure prominently in local commemorations at Northern Cheyenne. These commemorations were usually planned and implemented by particular family groups, military societies, or other sectors of the community and frequently drew criticism from others.

As an origin story for the reservation itself, Little Wolf and Dull Knife's journey north is the single most widely referenced nineteenth-century event at Northern Cheyenne. It is commemorated through two annual tribal holidays, including the January 9 Fort Robinson Outbreak, a site in Nebraska where Dull Knife's group was imprisoned and made a daring break for freedom, and the April 1 homecoming of Little Wolf's group. Imagery from a well-known 1873 photo of Dull Knife and Little Wolf appears in numerous venues, and the letterhead stationery of the Northern Cheyenne Tribe lists their names with the phrase: "Out of defeat and exile they led us back to Montana and won our Cheyenne homeland that we will keep forever." The local tribal college is named in honor of Dull Knife.

In addition to these institutionalized references, mentions of the epic journey north are made in a variety of social contexts and testify to their continuing persuasive force. For example, tribal members who have continued to advocate against recurrent proposals to mine reservation coal have underscored the need to protect the lands that their ancestors fought so hard to establish (see for instance Grossman [2005]). Tribal members who have organized an annual youth relay run from the site of the 1879 outbreak from Fort Robinson make the case that recollecting this journey reminds Northern Cheyenne youth that values of perseverance and courage are still relevant today. The motivational power of such moral claims was also evident during a candlelight walk through Lame Deer commemorating the outbreak that I attended in 1995, where an older woman slipped on the icy roads during the walk and was quickly helped by those around her. In the speeches afterward, several community leaders remarked that this display of aid should remind all present that a fundamental value of helping one another remains essential to being Northern Cheyenne, even while some community members now invest their time and energy in destructive social conflicts. Similar calls to maintain and strengthen an ethic of connection and aid in local social life are also evident in commentary in recent Northern Cheyenne activism for national recognition of their military victory at the 1876 Battle of the Rosebud (known to Cheyennes as the "Battle Where the Girl Saved Her Brother").

While the values of perseverance or caring for other Cheyennes are not usually openly challenged in these activities, controversies frequently arise when speakers explicitly link historical references to contemporary community issues or problems. Representations of gender roles and relations in accounts of the journey north serve as one example. While Dull Knife and Little Wolf are the major leaders associated with these events in both Cheyenne and non-Native accounts, others on record included Wild Hog, Tangle Hair (Powell 1969:198), and a young woman in Little Wolf's band who began having visions that are said to have guided the people (Powell 1969:209).[6] She is sometimes called Northern Walking Woman by present-day Cheyennes, and by the 1990s some community members were advocating for greater recognition of her role. As further evidence of the persuasive power that historical references can wield in local social life, many did so in an effort to assert a precedent for women's leadership in the tribe, and to then advocate for support for female candidates who were currently running for elected offices in tribal government.[7] Changing gender roles and relations have generated considerable local debate since the 1970s (see part II), however, and have fueled ongoing controversies about whether and how women should occupy formal political roles.

Controversies also arise when event organizers link historical commemoration with healing from past collective trauma. These activities pick up on broader trends that define historical trauma as a root cause of many contemporary problems in indigenous communities that can be healed through new forms of knowledge about past events (e.g., Duran and Duran 1995).[8] One Northern Cheyenne man has been instrumental in organizing and implementing the Spiritual Run for school-age youth at the site of the Fort Robinson Outbreak mentioned above. The group travels to the site on the January date of the event and approximates the journey undertaken by the survivors by running the 400 miles back to the reservation in relay style, taking breaks as needed in support vans. As public statements by the organizer describe, the primary goal of these practices is to promote a sense of responsibility for self and others, respect for the commitment and perseverance of their ancestors, experience with problem-solving skills, and a greater connection to the earth that is especially needed by youth at risk for serious consequences from substance abuse or other contemporary problems in reservation life. Other comments by the organizer and many participants with whom I have spoken emphasize how the act of running in the cold and along the same path as their ancestors produces a powerfully embodied form of historical knowledge. Activists responsible for establishing the Sand Creek Massacre site as a national historic site, described above, have similarly convened what they term a multigenerational "healing run" as an annual event to raise community awareness and support for their efforts, and in 2008 further undertook a Sand Creek Massacre Spiritual Healing Run for youth that spanned from the massacre site to Denver's city/county administration building.

Both of these sets of activities were viewed positively by numerous tribal members that I asked, with many expressing considerable respect for the time and energy devoted by the organizers and affirming the value of the historical education that they are providing. Yet many people were also critical of what they felt was partisanship that resulted in participation in the events primarily by selected kin groups, military society members, or others socially connected to the organizers. Many saw these divisions as evidence of the damages of colonization and noted the irony here, given that both efforts explicitly aim to help their participants heal from these historical legacies. More specific comments about the organizers and how they conduct themselves in family or public life, and about whether and how their upbringing included the degree of historical or ritual knowledge that they seemed to claim in organizing and implementing these events, often followed. Critics thereby took issue with the cultural identity and social authority of event organizers, evaluating them by locally prominent standards such as whether or not they possessed a conflict-reducing demeanor, pursued nonpartisan agendas, and had access to legitimate sources of historical and spiritual knowledge.

These brief examples illustrate how layers of moral commentary can emerge when Northern Cheyenne community members link historical references to contemporary social problems on the reservation.

These examples also indicate how references to both conflict reduction and spirituality figure prominently in this rhetoric. Local traditions of prophecy by the culture hero Sweet Medicine situate current community problems such as open conflict among tribal members and breaches of ritual protocol within a broader cosmology.

Prophecy and the Politics of Tradition

Sweet Medicine's teachings and prophecies were widely recorded in early ethnographies about the Cheyennes and continue to be mentioned frequently both at formal events and in informal discussions and debates about local issues of the day. With the loss of freedom and the imposition of radical changes to their lifeway in the late nineteenth century, the Northern Cheyennes were faced with interpreting what was happening and why. Many Cheyennes died from disease and violence in the tumultuous decades of warfare and dislocation just prior to the reservation's establishment. Poverty, malnutrition, and limited medical resources in the early reservation years brought continuing population losses through the 1920s (Moore 1999; see also Campbell 1989). Federal policies through the 1920s emphasized reforming Native economies, social organization, religions, and systems of governance by force to match those of non-Natives (Wilkins and Lomawaima 2002). As a result, the Northern Cheyennes were heavily pressured to take up infeasible economic pursuits such as small-scale farming, to send their children away to government- and missionary-run boarding schools, and to convert to Christianity while additional federal policies criminalized their local religious practices and forms of governance.

Many tribal members' accounts recorded during this time emphasized how these upheavals had resulted from broader disruptions in the order of the cosmos. Powell documents that many Northern Cheyennes in the late nineteenth century emphasized that there had been serious troubles with the two key sacred objects maintained by the tribe. The Sacred Arrows were captured in battle by the Pawnees in 1830, and in 1874 a dispute over succession erupted regarding the key ritual role of Keeper of the Sacred Buffalo Hat such that "the wife of the temporary Keeper . . . in a fit of anger, ripped a horn from Esevone [the Sacred Buffalo Hat]" (Powell 1969:38–39). By this logic, defeat stemmed from Cheyenne failures to properly care for these sacred objects in accordance with the teachings of Sweet Medicine and Erect Horns.

While superficially similar to popular Euro-American colonial narratives of the moral inferiority of Native peoples, these accounts differ strikingly in how they construct non-Natives not as powerful actors, but more as passive beneficiaries of Cheyenne error. They testify to the power of distinctive local perceptions of the new social order, and to the continuing vitality of local cosmologies and ritual practices, as the reservation era began.

Sweet Medicine's prophecies also seem to have powerfully shaped Northern Cheyenne interpretations of early reservation life and situate late nineteenth-century events in a much broader cosmological and historical framework. While ethnographers offer different accounts of these statements, all generally agree that Sweet Medicine predicted the coming of the horse, the war-oriented buffalo-hunting lifeway, the coming of Euro-Americans, the replacement of buffalo meat with the meat of white men's cattle as a dietary staple for the tribe, and, perhaps most importantly, the questionable future of the Cheyenne people. As Moore records:

> When you get toward the end, your people will begin to gray very young, and you will come to marry even your own relatives. You will reach a point where you will be ashamed of nothing, and you will act as if you were crazy.
>
> You will soon find among you a people who have hair all over their faces, and whose skin is white, and when that time comes, you will be controlled by them. The white people will be all over the land, and at last you will disappear. (1999:197–198)

Powell records a slightly different version, slightly less bleak in tone in that it emphasizes the importance of maintaining Sweet Medicine's teachings: "Before I die I have something to tell you. Now, my people, you must not forget what I am telling you today. You must not forget all that I have told you and taught you. When I am dead, you must come together often, and talk about these things. When you do this, always call my name." Yet this account also ends with the same statement as the previous one: "The white people will be all over the land; and at last you will disappear" (1969:466).

Grinnell recorded a version of the prophecies from White Bull, a well-known Northern Cheyenne healer and spiritual leader more widely known as Ice, in the early reservation years:

Those people will wander this way. You will talk with them. They will give you things like isinglass [i.e., things that flash or reflect the light, mirrors] and something that looks like sand that will taste very sweet. But do not take the things they give you. . . . Perhaps they will not listen to what you say to them, but you will listen to what they say to you. They will be people who do not get tired, but who will keep pushing forward, going, going all the time. They will keep coming, coming. They will try always to give you things, but do not take them. At last I think that you will take the things that they offer you, and this will bring sickness to you. These people do not follow the way of our great-grandfather. They follow another way. They will travel everywhere, looking for this stone which our great-grandfather put on the earth in many places. . . . [You will come to eat cattle instead of buffalo.] When you skin them, the flesh will jerk, and at last you will get this same disease. At last something will be given to you, which, if you drink it, will make you crazy. . . . [You will come to ride horses and travel far.] From that time you will act very foolishly. . . . You will be very foolish. You will know nothing. . . . You people will change: in the end of your life in those days you will not get up early in the morning; you will never know when day comes; you will lie in bed; you will have disease, and will die suddenly; you will all die off. At last those people will ask you for your flesh [your children] . . . but you must say "No." They will try to teach you their way of living. . . . those that they take away will never know anything. . . . They will tear up the earth, and at last you will do it with them. When you do, you will become crazy,[9] and will forget all that I am now teaching you. (1972b: 379–381)

While clearly echoing the versions cited above, this account also makes specific references to key problems in early reservation life such as the widespread health problems of this era, the increasing availability of alcohol, the forced assimilation policy of sending Native children away to boarding schools, and the plow-based farming and/or mining practices of American settlers.

By affirming the ongoing relevance of Cheyenne beliefs and ritual practices from the time of Sweet Medicine, yet also not defining exactly when or how the ultimate fate of the Cheyennes will be realized, these prophecies offer a robust rhetorical framework for interpreting contemporary problems through comparison to a past era. Their discursive legacies are numerous. While all versions of the prophecies predict a bleak future, for example, like other local historical references that emphasize the value of perseverance in the face of seemingly insurmountable odds, many Northern Cheyennes also seem to view them as calling for the Cheyennes to resist this fate as long as possible.

The push and pull of more fatalistic and more inspirational readings of the prophecies is evident in a variety of ethnohistorical and ethnographic materials (e.g., Stands in Timber and Liberty 1998; Weist 1978). Stands in Timber's oral history generally seems to call for the Cheyennes to preserve general cultural orientations advocated by Sweet Medicine, such as a calm and conflict-reducing demeanor, even as other specific practices that he brought to the people are no longer feasible under current conditions. Statements by tribal historian Bill Tallbull in the 1990s voiced similar themes, as in this comment to students during an ethnobotany class that I attended at the tribal college in 1995: "The old people in my day talked a lot about Sweet Medicine's prophecies. The future did not look good. There was no reason to argue. They sat quietly and tried to sustain their physical and spiritual well-being. Stayed away from the crowds, like at powwows and ballgames. Stayed home. Didn't take sides, in tribal politics. Prayed for everybody." These comments articulate the proper course of action under chaotic and difficult conditions as a dignified removal from this-worldly life, with an introspective focus on personal and collective survival. Like much of Stands in Timber's commentary, they also highlight animosity between tribal members as a key source of destruction for the Cheyennes. In offering specific depictions of which behaviors were destructive, yet also noting more constructive courses of action, the story's message does not seem to be one of giving up and accepting fate.

Indeed, I have found that fatalistic readings of Sweet Medicine's prophecies seemed far less prevalent on the reservation than more inspirational ones. Exceptions include Kathy, a woman born in the 1960s. I was present when she was visiting Mary, a female peer and neighbor, and the conversation turned to spiritual practices. As we were all aware, Mary was actively involved in running her own sweat lodge, fasting, and attending peyote meetings, while Kathy was not. Kathy explained why with reference to Sweet Medicine. As she said, her grandfather told her that Cheyenne ways were powerful but had become "no good any more." He explained how Sweet Medicine said that Cheyenne ways would disappear, and he said that this time had already come—otherwise, "Why are so many people fighting and marrying their cousins?" With the old ways gone, her grandfather felt that Christianity provided the best new way for the Cheyennes to lead a good life. Out of respect for him, Kathy said, she follows Christianity alone. A few weeks later, I mentioned to Mae, an elder who was well known for her experience with and knowledge of Cheyenne ceremonial practices, that I had heard that some Cheyennes believed that the end prophesied by Sweet Medicine had already come. She seemed surprised. "A few people are marrying their relatives, it is starting to happen," she allowed—but for the rest of the conversation then emphasized the need to maintain Cheyenne language and spiritual practices and described the work that she was doing (teaching her children, mentoring others in the community) toward this end. By her reckoning, the end may be near but is not yet upon the Cheyennes, leaving room for hope and continued cultural preservation—a sensibility that might best be termed one of guarded inspiration.

The prophecies' continuing motivational force is also evident in how frequently people use them to authorize points and positions in discussions of key political issues facing the community. Commentary by both actual and would-be political leaders on the reservation often mentions Sweet Medicine. (New communication technologies have facilitated this process, in fact, as in the 2000s when a tribal government website was constructed and the early ethnographic recording of Ice's version by George Bird Grinnell was reprinted in the October 2006 newsletter posted there.) References to the prophecies also figure in the recurrent local political debates about developing reservation coal. As in the 1970s, new proposals for coal development in subsequent decades have sparked opposition. By 2000, both activist and broader community attention focused not only on mining but also on the extraction of coal bed methane. This water-intensive method of extracting the gas from coal seams was already under way in areas surrounding the reservation and was generating serious concerns about downstream pollution of the Tongue River and other waterways on reservation lands.

In conversations during the 1990s some anti-coal activists specifically referenced Sweet Medicine's prophecies, saying that he had told the Cheyennes that they would come upon a "black stone" in the ground that they should leave alone. Such references seemed generally aimed at legitimating their aims, as well as at motivating others to join in the cause. These claims met with varied responses, however, as some community members agreed, while others took issue, making comments to me such as, "I have never heard that as part of the prophecies." Recall that multiple versions of the prophecies circulate; the one that Grinnell recorded from Ice (see chapter 2) did mention non-Native pursuits of a stone in the earth, but did not specify its color. Some critics of this claim were simply more supportive of coal development than the activists.

Indeed, the fall of 2006 witnessed an unprecedented reversal of recent political history, when the voting public at Northern Cheyenne affirmed a proposal to mine reservation coal reserves. During the preceding summer, I had witnessed several conversations about the upcoming vote. Some people said that their frustration with decades of continuing poverty was leading them to support the mining measure, while others continued to feel that the impact on environmental and cultural integrity was simply too great. The same election included the defeat of a proposal to develop coalbed methane, however, suggesting that anticoal activism has continued to impact local decision making. It is unclear whether the political efficacy of anti-coal activists' historical claims has lessened in recent years or whether changing demographics in who votes, shifting political fortunes of particular individuals on either side, or other factors shaped the outcomes of this particular election. What is clear from these events is that Sweet Medicine's prophecies remain an important reference point in local commentary and debate about contemporary social issues. The resulting debates also highlight the lack of consensus that surrounds claims about the content of the prophecies, however, as well as about what it means to be Cheyenne according to Sweet Medicine.

Often community members who make claims about prereservation eras of Cheyenne history, and especially the teachings of Sweet Medicine, describe these as "tradition," a term that at Northern Cheyenne as elsewhere connotes a sense of timelessness and continuity. Yet the prophecies themselves clearly recognize that past practices must be adapted to the changes imposed by colonization, charting space for considerable debate about exactly what elements of past lifeways can and should be carried forward under current conditions. Moreover, as Dole and Csordas (2003) describe for contemporary residents of the Navajo Reservation, what is "traditional" is frequently understood in multiple ways by people from different generations, areas of residence, educational levels, and so forth in contemporary reservation communities. In such contexts *tradition* is a term invested with moral meanings in response to current conditions and agendas, and these meanings are multiple rather than constituting a simply or easily shared "culture."

All human communities face the task of figuring ways to manage their localized diversity, and doing so is often essential for developing effective collective responses to social problems. Yet at Northern Cheyenne this task is complicated by the ways in which powerful local rhetorical conventions like Sweet Medicine's prophecies can raise the moral intensity of debates about both cultural identity and social authority, enabling claims that only certain ways of thinking and behaving are "traditional" and that anyone who disagrees is facilitating the dismal collective fate that the prophecies foretell. The resulting debates themselves can spark further layers of criticism, as many point out that conflict reduction is a key local value advocated by Sweet Medicine. Occasions when conflicts arise among ritual leaders on the reservation help to illustrate the social dynamics of these claims and counterclaims.

Conflicts are not uncommon during the planning of collective ceremonies like Sun Dances at Northern Cheyenne, and accounts of them are widely discussed in the community. While I cannot speak to how accurately these accounts depict the actual relationships among ceremonial people, conversations among community members often report that irreconcilable differences in understandings of proper ceremonial protocol arose, in which people on competing sides challenged the cultural identity and social authority of one another (e.g., "Where did he learn that? He says his grandfather raised him, but he spent most of his time at boarding school before his grandfather died, so how did he learn it from him?").

During some years, no consensus can be reached, and two or three separate Sun Dances are held. Some community members describe these conflicts as deeply troubling, and as evidence for how far the Cheyennes have departed from the unity of the past and violated Sweet Medicine's teachings. As a result, some avoid attending any Sun Dance with known major conflicts in its planning or implementation, saying that going forward with such rituals taps into powerful forces in ways that may actually create and perpetuate further troubles for the community. A broader critique of increasing diversity among tribal members is visible in some of this commentary, which constructs a moral center occupied by "really traditional" Northern Cheyennes whose efforts are being undermined by others who do not have the proper knowledge or comportment to belong to this select group.

Yet others see continuing value in Sun Dances and other collective rituals that is unaffected by conflict among ritual leaders. When more than one Sun Dance is held, they simply choose which one they feel most comfortable attending that year. Some even attend more than one.[10] Many who adopt this approach justify their actions with historical reference themselves, saying that diversity in understandings of protocol and practice have long legacies in Cheyenne ritual activities. From this perspective, the public conflict among ritual practitioners may be new, but their diversity of perspectives is not.

While the notion that there are multiple legitimate ways to be Cheyenne is also evident in the community, claims that some people are more genuinely Cheyenne than others are very prominent in local social life. People use a variety of different markers to evaluate who is "really" Cheyenne. Knowing and respecting one's kin carries great weight for some; conducting oneself in a congenial manner counts most for others, as does having completed an appropriate series of achievements in local ritual practices and so forth. Such claims are also made with varying intensity, often achieving the greatest rhetorical force when linked with the narrower definitions of *tradition*.

While varying in form and intensity, the rhetoric that only some community members are "real" Cheyennes broadly echoes the major non-Native interpretive frameworks and institutional practices that are imposed daily on reservation residents, many of which characterize contemporary diversity among the Northern Cheyennes as new, unexpected, and/or pathological. These non-Native interpretations reflect broader ideologies that clearly misrecognize Northern Cheyenne diversity, in the sense of adopting a highly selective view that obscures the interpretive and political-economic pressures that have both produced this diversity and shaped how it is understood (Bourdieu 1990). As such, while local rhetorics such as Sweet Medicine's prophecies have their own origins and social consequences, the constant presence of non-Native ideologies in the local cultural landscape may well reinforce how they posit highly exclusive definitions of what it means to be Northern Cheyenne.

Misrecognizing Diversity

As in other colonial contexts, the imposition of new administrative institutions in the reservation era has rested on the surveillance and monitoring of the Cheyenne population. Practices of taking censuses, allocating economic aid, enforcing legal penalties, schooling children, and providing health care have changed over time as U.S. federal policy and public sentiment have shifted. Yet all have continually involved incorporating Cheyennes into administrative rubrics that reflect the perspectives and interests of non-Natives, including the convenience of imposed definitions of tribal membership that imply that to be Northern Cheyenne does or should mean something fairly uniform. Closer reading of ethnographic and ethnohistorical materials, however, suggests that gender, kin groups, generation/age, and class differences have characterized most, if not all, eras in Northern Cheyenne history. In the reservation era these have been joined by growing differences in educational achievement, religion, language use, and kinship networks. The scope and nature of this diversity have been recurrently overlooked or pathologized by the priorities enacted through the agencies that administer reservation life, however.

To enact more administratively convenient social identities, the forced assimilation policies in the early reservation years involved constructing a system of family lines based upon Anglo-style surnames. To regulate distribution of treaty rights and the application of federal policies, these policies also introduced a system of tribal enrollment based on degree of Cheyenne "blood." This system reflected the rising popularity of biology as a tool to authorize social inequalities, as embodied by Euro-American investments in "racial science" in the eighteenth and nineteenth centuries (e.g., Stepan 1982). It departed significantly, however, from local practices of flexibility in recognizing tribal membership based on where and with whom one resided, and enhancing tribal numbers through adoption and intermarriage with members of other tribes. Moreover, the implementation of the new bio-bureaucratic system was riddled with inaccuracies. Northern Cheyenne children commonly resided with relatives other than their parents for periods of time, for example, and as a result census takers sometimes gave different surnames to children who had the same biological mother and father (Marquis 1978).

Blood quantum also produced new social categories of "full-blood" and "mixed blood" or "half-breed" that rapidly gained local cultural significance, and by the 1920s these were visibly implicated in political and interpersonal conflicts on the reservation (e.g., Marquis 1978:180). While descendance replaced blood quantum requirements for enrollment at Northern Cheyenne in the 1960s,[11] degrees of blood and/or evidence of direct ancestry remain prevalent in the administration of membership throughout Native American communities in the United States today (Garroutte 2003). At Northern Cheyenne, claims about blood and enrollment are frequently made in local debates about cultural identity and social authority.

In addition to these imposed social categories, other federal policies have produced new dimensions of diversity in Northern Cheyenne experiences. Relocation programs after World War II encouraged Native Americans on reservations to move to urban areas, and many Northern Cheyennes participated. These decades also witnessed heavy pressures from non-Native institutions to place children of unwed Cheyenne mothers up for adoption by non-Natives, as well as pressure from Christian missionaries who linked some of the best available educational opportunities for Northern Cheyenne children to living off the reservation with non-Native families. These practices created a segment of tribal members with little to no reservation experience, some of whom later returned to participate in community life as teenagers or adults. As a result, kinship networks continue to orient social life at Northern Cheyenne by structuring where many people live, with whom they socialize, and patterns of economic support and reciprocity; but the scope and workings of kinship ties also vary considerably by individuals and kin groups.

Distinct religious affiliations also soon marked new dimensions of diversity in the community, although these have shifted significantly over time. Pressures to convert to Christianity accompanied the criminalization of Native religious practices such as the Sun Dance in the early reservation era, and Catholic and Mennonite missionaries soon arrived. Yet outlawed practices persisted in some sectors of the community, and the peyote church (Native American Church) was embraced by a number of Northern Cheyenne families starting in the 1890s. Creative combinations of multiple beliefs and practices are not uncommon today, and in recent decades the Catholic and Mennonite churches have especially tended to acknowledge and support this trend. By the 1960s additional Christian denominations gained local popularity, including Lutheran, Baptist, Mormon, Jehovah's Witness, and Pentecostal. The more evangelical groups have offered greater opportunities for Northern Cheyennes to join the clergy than have the other sects but have also generally shown a stronger tendency to denounce participation in Northern Cheyenne ritual and Native American Church activities.

Variation in abilities to speak and understand Cheyenne also marks important social differences in the community. Generations of community members who experienced abuse for speaking Cheyenne in government- and church-run schools from the 1890s to the 1960s sometimes chose to protect their own children by having them learn only English. By the 1950s concerns about declining Cheyenne language use were evident in some sectors of the community, and contemporary Northern Cheyennes commonly note that even many fluent speakers today use newer forms and do not know the "old" version of Cheyenne. By the 1970s, researchers began documenting the decline in the proportion of tribal members fluent in the Cheyenne language (Straus 1976; Ward and Wilson 1989; Weist 1977). Numerous efforts toward language revitalization have been implemented in response, through school-based programs and immersion camps.[12] The ability to speak Cheyenne is often implicated in debates about cultural identity and social authority— although as with other markers of identity, different people prioritize language use quite differently. For example, some, but not all, community members consider the ability to pray in Cheyenne essential for legitimate participation in the Sun Dance, fasting, and other ritual practices.

Finally, educational opportunities have also introduced important dimensions of difference and have shifted across generations in concert with changing federal policies and Native activism for greater local control of schooling. Access to quality education has remained a persistent problem, with many generations experiencing high dropout rates (see Ward 2005). At Northern Cheyenne, as throughout the United States, educational achievement is linked with economic opportunity, yet given the general limitations on employment and business opportunities on the reservation, underemployment is also widespread and many of the most highly educated local residents seek better opportunities off the reservation.

While examples of how new social identities have emerged as the result of federal policies and institutional practices are relatively easy to describe, local ways of responding to differences among tribal members are more difficult to chart. But the form and/or political force of local rhetorics that make the most exclusionary claims about who is "really" Northern Cheyenne may stem at least in part from their similarity to prominent non-Native narratives of U.S. history. Many of these frame the conquest of Native America as inevitable, if not justified, and do so through the continual and pervasive retelling of a story that emplots Native American history as a decline from a golden age. This story widely recirculates through textbooks, museums, movies, and various ways of "playing Indian" through summer camp activities, toys, and reenactment events (Deloria 1998). In North America as in many colonial contexts (Asad 1995; Comaroff and Comaroff 1992; Said 1978), such ideas often serve to naturalize persistent inequalities between colonizer and colonized. While Northern Cheyennes also construct a trajectory of loss through rhetorics such as Sweet Medicine's prophecies, these local claims can take a variety of forms, can inspire an array of actions, and generally challenge rather than justify the power inequalities between Native and non-Native societies. Yet when local rhetorics are used to cast "real" Northern Cheyenne identity in narrow terms that exclude major segments of the community, their form and effects coincide with those of prominent non-Native discourses and practices.

The impact of such non-Native perspectives may be especially marked in regions like the Great Plains. Northern Cheyennes and other Plains peoples have been subjected to an especially heavy dose of stereotyped "Indian" imagery. The nomadic equestrian lifeway of Native peoples on the nineteenth-century Great Plains serves as an icon of "Indians" both within North America (Kilpatrick 1999) and globally (Penny 2006), and this imagery supports narratives of Native history as disruption of a coherent and stable lifeway. Closer readings of both classic and lesser-known ethnographic and ethnohistorical accounts, however, provide evidence for ongoing change and significant social diversity among the Cheyennes across the different eras of their collective history.

Revisiting "Plains Indian" Imagery

One of the most widely read ethnographic accounts of the Cheyennes depicts their nineteenth-century buffalo-hunting lifeway as a coherent cultural "climax" (Hoebel 1978:12) that was then disrupted by military defeat and reservation life. This narrative of decline overlooks the considerable evidence for long-standing histories of adaptation and internal diversity among the Cheyennes, however, and emphasizes non-Native power by implying that the only significant diversity in Cheyenne priorities, perspectives, and actions came in response to Euro-American colonization.

Closer reading of ethnographic and ethnohistorical accounts suggests otherwise. For example, buffalo hunting did not completely dominate the nineteenth-century Cheyenne economy but was situated within a more complicated historical shift in subsistence strategies. Moore's meticulous reconstruction of historical transformations in Cheyenne economy, social structure, and political institutions (1987, 1999) describes the ancestors of the Cheyennes as members of diverse Algonquian groups, who coalesced into a unified tribe calling themselves Tsitsistas[13] by the early 1700s (1999:146). Moore (1987) cites evidence of four different bands sharing a central settlement by this time and suggests that in the early eighteenth century, the group made the decision to apply one band name to the group as a whole (1999:146), perhaps because the Tsitsistas group held a position of some dominance or perceived stability relative to others.

Both Moore's account and Weist's extensive ethnohistory (1977) emphasize that the people arrived on the Plains after an early era of food foraging with an emphasis on small game, followed by a long period practicing horticulture along riverbanks, while living in earth lodge villages fortified with earthen walls. The end of the eighteenth century found the Tsitsistas combining horticulture with hunting on the Middle Missouri River, a major trade center on the Plains in this era. Here they acquired both horses and guns and soon moved westward into the Black Hills region, where they began hunting buffalo more intensively and came to occupy a lucrative niche, mediating the trade of buffalo and other items from the Plains, produce from the Missouri River tribes, and goods from Euro-American trading posts.

Yet the buffalo hunting trade did not completely supplant earlier economic strategies or associated cultural institutions. As Iron Teeth (1834–1928), in a narrative recorded by physician and attentive amateur ethnographer Thomas Marquis in the 1920s, describes: "We planted corn every year when I was a little girl in the Black Hills. With sharpened sticks we punched holes in the ground, dropped in the grains of corn, and went hunting all summer. When the grass died we returned and gathered the crop. But the Pawnees and Arikaras got to stealing or destroying our growing food, so we had to quit the plantings. We got into the way then of following all the time after the buffalo and other herds" (1978:54–55). Grinnell cites evidence for continued planting through 1865 (1972a:251–253). Some references also indicate that not all Cheyennes cared much for the new buffalo-centered foodways, with Powell citing a nineteenth-century Cheyenne woman who recalled "her grandmother's knowledge of songs praising the old times 'when they lived on fishes and fowls, and had not to eat this nauseating buffalo meat'" (1969:19–20)! Powell documents that sacred ears of corn were still carried with the tribe until they were destroyed by American soldiers in the mid-1870s and records the persistence of a corn dance healing ritual involving women dancers through the Plains years and even into the early reservation years (1969:28–29).

Moreover, rather than affirming popular imagery of a society clearly and coherently oriented around warfare, many ethnographies document how high degrees of ambivalence about violence were codified in nineteenth-century Cheyenne life. Accounts emphasize how in giving them the Sacred Arrows, Sweet Medicine admonished the Tsitsistas to interact with one another peaceably and noted that chiefs in particular should behave as exemplars of emotionally controlled, benevolent behavior. Numerous sources document how nineteenth-century Cheyenne chiefs were esteemed for calm and measured responses to even the most trying of life's difficulties (e.g., the murder of a son, betrayal by a spouse) (Grinnell 1972a; Hoebel 1978; Stands in Timber and Liberty 1998). Various sources also record that war leaders and society men were criticized by their peers and the community at large for being too "mean," for example, if they seemed to take pleasure in delivering punishments when policing tribal members (see Llewelyn and Hoebel 1941:121,145), suggesting a broader cultural concern with constraining the exercise of aggression. Moreover, Sweet Medicine taught that if one tribal member murdered another, then the Arrows would become flecked with blood and must be ritually renewed. The antagonist was also exiled for four years, and upon his[14] eventual return was culturally conceptualized as suffering from an irreversible process of inward decay that barred him from full participation in social and ritual life. The Sacred Buffalo Hat tipi also served a peace-keeping function, creating a neutral ground during disputes with the belief that no one who entered the lodge could be harmed (e.g., Powell 1969:183).

Still further cultural alternatives to the calm/chiefly and tough/warrior demeanors are evidenced among nineteenth-century Cheyenne women. Some women's activities involved more open forms of emotional expression than were conventional for men, and seem to have been positively valued for their capacity to inspire compassion.[15] Llewellyn and Hoebel describe how the decision to allow an exiled murderer to return articulated a powerful cultural value placed upon rehabilitation and was often made at the urging of the banished man's wife, who took responsibility for conveying the misery of the family's condition to tribal leaders (1941:133). Cheyenne women also played primary roles in the expression of grief at a close relative's death, expressed through a dramatic symbolic and material renunciation of social participation. The deceased's possessions were abandoned for any nonrelated tribal member to take, leaving the family dependent upon the generosity of other community members for the period of mourning. Women then cut their hair, slashed their arms and legs, and sometimes cut off one of their finger joints, to express the depth of their feeling and to solicit compassion from both the spirit and human worlds (Grinnell 1972b:196). These activities seem to have been accorded high esteem and even articulated tribal identity in some forums (e.g., in intertribal Plains Indian sign language, the sign for "Cheyenne" translates as "cut finger people").

Most accounts of nineteenth-century Cheyennes also suggest that gender organized social life through spheres of activity and experience that were often separate but complementary. Cheyenne women could gain prestige through their domestic skills (e.g., lodge raising, decorative arts like quillwork and beadwork), and also through maintaining chastity in their youth. While an emphasis on sexual modesty might reflect a gender-specific means of achieving honor in a society oriented around male war activities (cf. Abu-Lughod 1986), Cheyenne women seem to have held noteworthy power in the regulation not only of female but also of male sexual behavior. Llewellyn and Hoebel record that any man who attempted to transgress a young Cheyenne woman's chastity rope was asking for trouble from her female relatives, who might well gash his lodge or other of his property with knives (1941:177). Moreover, although menstrual and other taboos did circumscribe premenopausal women's involvement, the realm of nineteenth-century ritual practice seems to have afforded opportunities for both men and women. Both played valued roles in the major collective ceremonies,[16] and both could earn spiritual power through more spontaneous visions and dreams, often featuring an animal figure that instructed the dreamer (Stands in Timber and Liberty 1998:103–104). Cheyenne healers often received a calling to their art in this fashion and then sought technical instruction from an established practitioner. As Grinnell records, at any given time the tribe included approximately equal numbers of female and male healers (1972b:166), and many postmenopausal women practiced independently, while male healers could not practice without a female assistant (1972b:128–129).

Cheyenne women also wielded noteworthy influence in collective decision making. Grinnell notes that Cheyenne women may once have held formal positions in the chief's councils, and describes how in collective decision-making their "influence . . . can hardly be overestimated, and in the councils so frequently held, where only men spoke, this influence of the women was always felt" (1972a:156–157). At another point he emphasizes that "the women are the rulers of the camp. . . . If the sentiment of the women of the camp clearly points to a certain course as desirable, the men are quite sure to act as the women wish" (1972a:128–129). Later accounts by Stands in Timber and Liberty (1998:63) and Moore (1999:250) affirm that the motivational power of women's "gossip," or commentary about decisions and events affecting the community, had long been recognized in the deliberations and actions of tribal leaders. Postmenopausal women exercised this influence most intensively, potentially earning the status of "woman chief" within their kin groups and beyond (Moore 1999).

Popular imagery of male domination in Cheyenne life may unduly emphasize nineteenth-century changes to more established cultural patterns. Moore (1999) suggests that women's economic power had been substantial during the horticultural era, given their primary responsibility for food production. Origin stories describing the tribe's acquisition of corn feature powerful female protagonists, in a striking contrast to the male culture heroes of the buffalo-hunting era. Occasional instances of collective sexual violence against women by the military societies were also widely recorded by early ethnographers, who described them as anomalous practices that drew censure from many Cheyennes (Grinnell 1972a; Hoebel 1978; Llewellyn and Hoebel 1941). The increasing warfare of the mid-nineteenth century might have removed barriers and/or presented opportunities for more aggressive and violent Cheyenne men, at least in some sectors of the community.

These brief examples of ongoing adaptation, diversity, and debate in the nineteenth-century and earlier eras of Cheyenne history challenge the well-known narratives that position the buffalo-hunting era as one of exceptional cultural coherence or stability. Most of these details are not widely discussed among contemporary Northern Cheyennes that I know but are well known to tribal members who have more specialized historical knowledge. But even as the buffalo-hunting era also figures in the most prominent Northern Cheyenne imagery of their history, local social life does feature commentary that explicitly notes how Northern Cheyenne and non-Native understandings of this era are different. One man commented at a public workshop about domestic violence, for example, that Cheyenne men who glorify violence as part of their masculinity have uncritically absorbed messages about how to be Cheyenne from B movies rather than from local cultural history. As he elaborated, nineteenth-century Cheyenne men's primary responsibilities were to protect and provide for their families, and their roles as warriors served these priorities rather than being an end in themselves.

Health Concerns in Local Cultural Context

The local cultural landscape of the Northern Cheyenne Reservation features a distinctive historical consciousness, local claims that link historical experiences to contemporary problems, and politicized rhetorics about cultural identity that fuel debate about the authority and legitimacy of these claims. While the reservation community is clearly culturally distinct from the surrounding non-Native world, it is also composed of multiple local moral worlds, rather than constituting an easily definable, shared "culture."

How does this complex cultural environment shape local responses to health concerns such as alcohol use? Whether particular claims implicate alcohol more directly or tangentially in contemporary reservation problems, most commentary about drinking emphasizes how alcohol arrived as part of the Euro-American invasions of the Great Plains. "White man's water" is the English translation of the major Cheyenne term for alcohol, *vé?ho?e-mahpe,* which specifically refers to hard liquor, especially whiskey.[17] Ethnographic studies elsewhere in Native North America have demonstrated the significance of historical references for interpreting and responding to a wide range of health problems (Adelson 2000; Garro and Lang 1994; Schwarz 1995). Forced changes in lifeway, land losses and ecological damage, and lack of political autonomy figure prominently within the interpretive frameworks that connect experiences of colonization both to specific health problems and to generally threatened well-being. Yet making historical references can and does spark considerable debate in communities like Northern Cheyenne, and these controversies in turn provoke a range of responses. While many draw links between historical experience and current problems, to trace these links as due to errors or oversights in ritual practice suggests a very different solution than tracing them to conflict-producing demeanors or to language loss. The notion that Northern Cheyenne history has produced widespread emotional trauma encourages still another type of solution. These local theories about how historical experiences have shaped contemporary problems are not necessarily distinct in practice, either, but can be creatively combined as community members use and negotiate among them.

Health services on the reservation face special barriers to recognizing and accommodating these local complexities, given ongoing structural pressures to view social, cultural, and/or psychological diversity as a "problem" and needs to contend with uneven and limited resources. A pattern of sporadic and limited investment in health services was especially evident in Native North America through the mid-1950s (Davies 2001; Jones 2004), but even after the emergence of the federal Indian Health Service in 1954 and the gains of civil rights activism through the middle decades of the twentieth century, disparities in the quality of health care and in health outcomes have continued between Native Americans and the general U.S. population (Jones 2006; Kunitz 2000). Gathering information about local perspectives and needs, and using it as the basis for developing health programs, has generally remained a low priority. Federal resource investment in many communities has instead been oriented around interventions into perceived crises using therapies deemed to work in non-Native contexts. The following chapter takes a closer look at how Northern Cheyenne perspectives on drinking reflect the rhetorical strategies and cultural concerns described here, and how key responses within federally funded reservation health services have failed to accommodate these local complexities.

3

Contextualizing "White Man's Water"

For community members experiencing substance abuse problems on the Northern Cheyenne Reservation, the local federally funded health service system provides one central program. Recovery Center is located in the reservation's administrative center of Lame Deer. It is staffed primarily by Northern Cheyenne community members who have completed specialized training in chemical dependency counseling. By the 1990s, its programs for clients, local public workshops, and referrals to off-reservation inpatient treatment centers demonstrated a marked reliance on the concepts and practices drawn from the Twelve Steps of Alcoholics Anonymous.

Recovery Center services heavily emphasize, for example, the foundational Twelve Step idea that one needs to overcome the denial of how alcohol is impacting one's life in order to achieve sobriety, and the correlated notion that instead of habitually reacting by drinking, one needs to learn to experience and express emotions in new ways. One counselor noted how greater awareness of one's emotional experiences and reactions can support new behaviors, explaining, "We try to teach them about taking time to think—not just go from event to action. Then they can think of other ways to deal with a situation. A lot of people just react, without using that thinking process."

To support this more reflexive mode of experience, Recovery Center programs use numerous conventions established within Twelve Step meetings, such as encouraging clients to learn and use terms such as *alcoholic* to describe themselves, and to engage a variety of new terms for expressing emotion. Many activities especially focus on helping clients to identify painful emotions such as grief, shame, and anger, and to process these feelings through talking with counselors, sponsors, clients, or other supportive people.

Recovery Center clients who report feeling helped by these practices emphasize how talking has indeed facilitated their coming to better

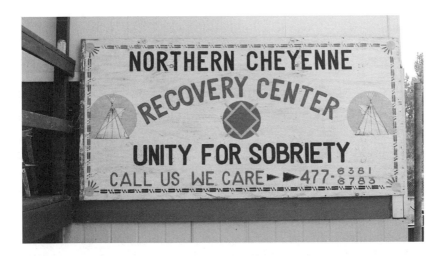

Figure 5. This handpainted sign for the Recovery Center includes the symbol for the Northern Cheyenne Tribe, the morning star, at its center. Photo by the author.

terms with painful experiences, especially those that generated powerful emotions such as grief, hatred, or shame. Louise (born in the 1950s) described how learning about "abandonment" helped her to comprehend and better manage the power of grief:

> Going to treatment was one of the best things I ever done for myself, because I learned a lot that I never knew before. I grieved for my grandmother for years, and I didn't even know it. I stayed with her more than with my parents [when I was growing up]. I used to still dream about my grandmother, and every time I'm just about ready to touch her or hug her or something, I'd wake up and I'd feel sad, really sad, where I'd start crying. I felt that abandonment and—well, you see I didn't know all these words 'til I went to treatment. Talking about it helped. Then when I dreamt about her, I got to hug her. And I woke up really peaceful. I didn't cry anymore.

Yet many other Northern Cheyennes who come to Recovery Center find these approaches to be quite alienating. At one of the many Family Day prevention education sessions at Recovery Center that were open to the public, participants received a page with approximately 50 different emotion terms, in English, with line drawings of faces to illustrate each. The facilitator of the session played a video, also in English and developed by Hazelden (a prominent recovery institute in Minnesota), that featured all-Anglo actors and was intended to illustrate how one could avoid unpleasant conflicts with family and friends by identifying and expressing one's emotions. She then asked for people's responses to the film, and the room was silent. In my experience, such silences were frequent at these types of sessions, unless the facilitator called on people or led a more structured response activity, such as asking each person present to select an emotion term to describe one of their own personal experiences. In nondirective interviews, many clients who attended these kinds of sessions reported feeling like they were in a school-like setting receiving information in ways that did not inspire their participation, and also feeling discomfort with the emphasis on disclosing their emotional experiences in front of a group. Many commented that they found it somewhat more helpful to see recovery films about Native communities, to hear more personal testimonies from Native counselors and community members, and for a significant minority, to attend sessions and meetings conducted in the Cheyenne language. Yet for many still, even these seemingly more "culturally appropriate" approaches that were periodically included in Recovery Center's services did not fully resolve strong feelings of discomfort about the modes of self-expression that are seen as essential to recovery within the Twelve Steps. As a result, many ultimately stopped coming to Recovery Center.

Feelings of discomfort and high dropout rates are certainly not uncommon in substance abuse or other mental health programs in any community. Yet on the Northern Cheyenne Reservation, Twelve Step concepts and practices clearly encounter and often conflict with local ethnopsychologies, or cultural conventions of emotional expression and self-presentation. For example, after attending a Recovery Center–sponsored community workshop in which a number of speakers used narrative forms conventionalized within Twelve Step recovery to tell tearful stories of their drinking days and journey to sobriety, Morris (born in the 1950s) commented:

> It is good that they express their feelings. You need to do that, to cry if you need to. But I look at that crying in public as self-pity—standing up there and crying into that microphone means that you are asking people to pity you. We have all been though hard times, so why should

I pity someone? In public, people should express their feelings in a story or another way—build them into something that other people can feel and appreciate. Just crying up there, it's like you haven't dealt with it. People don't want to see that; they want to see and appreciate how other people can take their pain and make it into something.

Whereas many Twelve Step adherents on the reservation take tears and other expressions of raw emotion as evidence of a progressive process toward self-transformation, Morris casts them as evidence of stagnation (i.e., one who "hasn't dealt with" their suffering) and as attempts to make unwarranted claims for sympathy. At Northern Cheyenne, as in other Northern Plains communities (cf. Anderson 2001; O'Nell 1996), some local understandings of the nature of personhood, social relations, and well-being cast "pity" as motivation for expressions of compassion and connection that affirm shared collective experiences (see also Straus 1977). Morris portrays Twelve Step–style claims as failing to engage this distinctive ethnopsychological perspective, however, instead eliciting a response of alienation and dismissal.

Twelve Step approaches to alcohol-related problems have therefore entered into a complex cultural environment at Northern Cheyenne that features different perceptions of whether and how drinking is problematic, as well as multiple modes of achieving sobriety. Disparate responses by community members feature rhetorics similar to those visible in broader local commentary about contemporary community problems, which often connect current troubles to past colonial injustice and violence. Yet community members voice divergent and competing perspectives on how to craft claims about the causes of problems, how to legitimate these claims, and how to advocate for particular courses of action in response. Debates about alcohol problems specifically highlight how diverse local ethnopsychological understandings of person, self, and emotion can figure within these conflicts.

Despite clear local debate and myriad expressions of alienation, however, programs based on Twelve Step therapies have been institutionalized for decades in the reservation's federally funded health services. Examining how that happened demonstrates that despite the multiple local meanings of drinking and sobriety at Northern Cheyenne and marked social and psychological diversity among community members, federally funded health programs face ongoing barriers to recognizing and accommodating these complexities.

While documenting local cultural understandings and uses of alcohol has been a mainstay of ethnographic research in the interdisciplinary field of alcohol studies, in Native North America these findings are often over-shadowed by conventional wisdom about "Indian drinking." Popular stereotypes that alcohol use by Native Americans is universal, inevitable, and incorrigible are so widespread that they often override ethnographic findings about localized variation in experiences, problems, and needs.

Alcohol in Native North America: Politics of Perception

Stereotyped ideas that "all Indians are drunks," "Indians just can't hold their liquor," and related claims have an extensive history in North America. While patterns of widespread, normative alcohol use on the Northern Cheyenne Reservation might initially seem to fit well with this imagery, a far more complicated story emerges from a closer look at when and how alcohol use became widespread in the community, who drinks, and when and how people stop drinking.

Alcohol was introduced to Native Americans within the context of an ideologically charged colonial encounter. With the exception of some groups in the Southwest who produced fermented beverages, Native North Americans do not seem to have manufactured alcoholic beverages prior to the introduction of both fermented and distilled forms by Europeans (Mail and McDonald 1980). Perceptions that Natives and Euro-Americans responded differently to alcohol were frequently recorded in European colonial and early American historical records (Calloway 1997; Mancall 1995). In particular, assumptions that Native drinking produced severe inebriation, violence, sexual license, and other social problems are documented among both Natives and non-Natives, as are concerns that Native drinking fueled the exploitation of Natives by Euro-American traders. As a result, beginning in the mid-1700s various European colonial powers in North America passed laws prohibiting the sale of alcohol to and/or use of alcohol by Native peoples. With the formation of the United States later that century, federal prohibition policies were upheld, remaining in place until 1952.

The widespread circulation of these concerns and their codification in law serve political purposes. Broad generalizations that being Native inherently includes a greater tendency to drink and/or to become inebriated fit well with colonial agendas of constructing a social hierarchy that positions non-Natives as superior to Natives (May 1994; Quintero 2001).

Denying the full moral worth of Native peoples supported broader colonial agendas of genocide and ethnocide, while portraying Native peoples as inherently vulnerable supported paternalistic ideas that colonial "protection" was required for Native survival (Berkhofer 1978; Dippie 1982). Numerous historical studies document how colonial records and subsequent popular perceptions enacted and reproduced stereotypes about "Indian drinking" by disregarding the clearly observable diversity and complexities of alcohol use among those classified as "Indian" (e.g., Abbott 1999). Ethnographic and epidemiological studies have offered reason to question claims that there are always categorical differences between alcohol use by Natives and non-Natives. Many find numerous similarities between the drinking practices of Natives and non-Natives who share numerous demographic features besides ethnic identity (Levy and Kunitz 1974), while others demonstrate the diversity of drinking rates, styles, and consequences for different Native communities (Beals et al. 2009; May 1994).

Studies that critically examine popular stereotypes about Native North Americans and alcohol have variously termed them the "drunken Indian stereotype" (Bird 1996) or "firewater myth" (Leland 1976). Why have these persisted in popular consciousness, despite considerable evidence to the contrary? A partial answer to this question lies in how stereotypes simplify and overgeneralize, effectively detracting attention from more complex and potentially troubling questions about what and who might be responsible for causing—and therefore, for remedying—alcohol-related problems.

For example, biological explanations hold that genetic and/or physiological factors cause Native Americans to metabolize alcohol differently than non-Natives. These explanations remain extraordinarily popular, despite the fact that considerable research has never substantiated them (Leland 1976; May 1994). As with the "thrifty gene" explanation for disproportionate rates of diabetes among Native Americans (Paradies et al. 2007) and the "virgin soil" explanation for early Native American mortality from infectious diseases (Jones 2003), such explanations may garner high levels of explanatory power in the absence of good evidence because they engage the broader cultural authority of biology and especially the late-twentieth-century fascination with genetics (Goodman et al. 2003), offering a tidy rationalization of health disparities that could otherwise raise thorny political questions about their social origins. While biological research is certainly needed, assumptions need to be replaced with more careful and accurate assessment of biological contributors to alcohol problems.[1]

Psychosocial explanations also very commonly accompany ideas about unique Native American susceptibilities to problems with alcohol. These maintain that Native Americans drink in response to the stresses of their disempowered position as colonized peoples, including cultural disruptions that have produced widespread experiences of confusion and anomie. As Waldram (2004) cogently argues, however, such theories also suffer from reductionism and inaccuracy, fueling stereotyped notions that all contemporary Native peoples are pathological, and continuing to focus attention on Native behavior as the central problem, even while they purport to attend to historical and social factors. Psychosocial explanations are most constructively viewed as possibilities that need to be examined through careful attention to personal and local community histories, rather than being globally presumed to apply clearly or equally to all Native peoples (Gone 2009; Medicine 2007).

These critiques of popular stereotypes call for multifactorial understandings of Native American alcohol use that can account for how drinking practices vary between and among Native individuals and communities. Works in the multidisciplinary field of alcohol studies have emphasized how some of the most-publicized, binge styles of drinking adopted by some Native Americans can be significantly explained by social and economic factors (e.g., Frank et al. 2000). Heavy drinking played a central role in the social and economic life of non-Natives on colonial frontiers. In the American West, for instance, heavy alcohol consumption was a major recreational pursuit of the trappers, traders, cowboys, railroad workers, and others who comprised the majority of early settlers.[2] Many observers have remarked upon the ways in which these settlers served as role models for some Native Americans who had close social contact with them (e.g., MacAndrew and Edgerton 1969). Others have noted that the policies of prohibition themselves have continually encouraged binge-drinking practices, in areas where these have been adopted, as a means of disposing of all available ill-gotten goods quickly (May 1994).

In addition to social learning and the effects of policy, powerful economic pressures sustained the liquor trade in Native America throughout the colonial era. Mancall (1995) emphasizes how alcohol continued to be an essential trade item in frontier economies even after prohibition policies were on the books. He describes a basic contradiction between the prohibition policies of settlements at colonial centers and the realities of life in peripheral areas. In essence, the practical exigencies of frontier life encouraged and facilitated Native behavior that was then perceived as inappropriate by those in colonial centers. As a result, an ongoing supply of alcohol generated continuing opportunities to include drinking in the wider-ranging impressions of Native inferiority that accompanied intensifying Euro-American colonial expansion.

Alongside such historical analyses, ethnographic studies have worked to challenge entrenched stereotypes by documenting the diversity and complexity of contemporary Native Americans' experiences with alcohol.[3] Many emphasize the need to consider local worlds of meaning as well as the politics of Native/non-Native relations when attempting to understand alcohol-related practices and problems (O'Nell and Mitchell 1996). Recent works have begun to focus less on how or why Native peoples drink, and more on how they stop drinking (e.g., Bezdek and Spicer 2006; Kunitz and Levy 1994; Medicine 2007; Quintero 2000; Spicer 2001). This emphasis arguably offers greater resistance to appropriation by the reductionistic biological and psychosocial explanations described above (see also Quintero 2001) and is also potentially of greater practical use to those who are working to promote sobriety in Native communities.

Medicine (2007) especially calls for ethnographers working with Native peoples to not simply focus on contemporary practices, perceptions and responses to drinking, but also include more diachronic perspectives on local community experiences with alcohol. Such approaches more effectively challenge generalizations about "drunken Indians," as well as reductionistic uses of theories of social learning and historical trauma. By enriching understanding of local cultural repertoires, tracing key themes in local perceptions and responses to alcohol over time and how they have interacted through changing conditions, such historical perspectives can also support efforts to best fit prevention and intervention efforts within local cultural realities. A brief history of Northern Cheyenne experiences with alcohol highlights the diversity of perspectives on alcohol within the community through different eras. It also illuminates ongoing disjunctures between these local realities and the responses to drinking-related health problems that have been institutionalized in reservation health services over time.

Northern Cheyennes: Early Encounters with Alcohol

Most sources suggest that drinking was generally limited to a few individuals and family groups on the Northern Cheyenne Reservation prior to the 1930s. The Cheyennes seem to have first encountered whiskey on the southern Plains in the 1830s, most notably at John Gantt's trading post on the Upper Arkansas River (Marquis 1978:54). Elderly community members told me that sustained access to alcohol came much later, when tribal members worked as scouts at Fort Keogh, Montana, in the 1880s. Drinking still remained relatively infrequent in the community for several subsequent decades. Both ethnographic and ethnohistorical sources suggest a fundamental ambivalence in Cheyenne responses to alcohol in this era: drinking tended to be viewed negatively when linked with interpersonal violence and conflict but was also positively linked with good times and celebration.

The classic ethnographic works about the Cheyennes include only scattered and generally undeveloped references to alcohol but affirm that drinking was relatively infrequent in the nineteenth century. Most portray it as a predominantly male activity that was frequently linked with the military societies. Llewellyn and Hoebel mention the resolution of a dispute involving the Kit Fox Society in the mid-nineteenth century, for example, in which horses were given to the Kit Foxes in restitution. They quote an informant as saying: "These men took them to a trader in a deal for a barrel of whiskey. Then they set up a feast and invited all the military clubs to a good binge. They had a good time and no harm was done" (1941:123). Stands in Timber's oral history also suggests that drinking and drunken behavior could serve as sources of entertainment. He tells one amusing story of a man named Buffalo Horn, who, after a bout of drinking in Miles City, chose to return to the base at Fort Keogh through an old riverbed. With inebriated prudence he chose to take off his clothes, lest they become soiled. He reached the other side, coated with muck and completely naked. Still mindful of propriety, he found some prayer cloths tied to a tree on the other side and fastened those on himself like a breechclout. As Stands in Timber continues: "And then he heard the bugle sound for suppertime. Everyone told how he came running across the flat as hard as he could go, with no clothes on and that cloth flying. He stopped at the end of the line with his feet together and his arms down straight, and that broke it up—there was no more roll call. They said the captain in charge nearly died laughing" (1998:231).

Various ethnographers also report that drinking was sometimes associated with violence, however, including homicides (e.g., Hoebel 1978:38; Grinnell 1972a:98–100) that often occurred in the aftermath of drinking-related sexual liaisons and resulting interpersonal conflicts (Grinnell 1972b:98–100; Llewellyn and Hoebel 1941:137). In perhaps the most well-known example, several sources describe how an alcohol-related homicide dealt a major, disorganizing blow to the chief's council in 1880. After helping to lead the epic journey back north, Little Wolf killed Starving Elk while under the influence of alcohol (Llewellyn and Hoebel 1941:84; Powell 1969:289–90). He lived in self-imposed exile until 1892, when other council and community members decided to renew the Council of Forty-four Chiefs. There was considerable debate over how to handle the fact that Little Wolf was living in exile for murder, as this meant that everything in his possession was defiled, but he was still in possession of an especially sacred chief's medicine bundle. Accounts vary as to what happened next (see Llewellyn and Hoebel 1941), but Stands in Timber describes how the chiefs coped with this contradiction by ritually renewing the bundle in an Arrow Renewal Ceremony (1998:48).

As a result of such events, records do indicate that some sectors of the community perceived drinking as a problem in this era. Stands in Timber describes how local efforts were made to curb drinking and its consequences in the early decades of reservation life, as a means of containing unwanted "trouble":

Sometimes the old Indians would fix a person who made trouble drinking, but they don't do it anymore. It happened once in Miles City when they had a big Stampede on the Fourth of July, around 1925. Red Water, one of the first educated Indians . . . was the troublemaker. He had gone to school at Haskell and was a top football player, and he got a fine place when he came back to the reservation. But he neglected it and lost it, and never used his education, and whenever he started drinking he wanted to fight. This time in Miles City he had been chasing everybody out of their camps and they got mad at him. Finally Wooden Leg threw him down and hog-tied him. He was a strong man, but it took some others to help him. They tied Red Water's hands and hung him up by the feet over the limb of a tree. His head almost touched the ground. He was there for several hours. At last somebody cut him loose. His face was all swelled up but he was all right, and he did not make any more trouble for a while. But he was always bad when he got drunk. (1998:276)

By linking Red Water's drinking to wasted potential, Stands in Timber's story seems to echo some versions of Sweet Medicine's prophecies, which describe a drink that will make the Cheyennes "crazy" and contribute to their ultimate disappearance. In noting that "fixing" Red Water in this fashion was only a temporary solution, Stands in Timber links alcohol use to personal pathology and social disruption. In observing that similar interventions are no longer practiced, he also seems to employ the broader rhetoric of decline from past to present that continues to figure so prominently in local commentary about current problems in reservation life.

Yet while alcohol clearly figured as a troubling problem in some local commentary in the early decades of reservation life, alternative perspectives are also evident. Llewellyn and Hoebel (1941) report that drunkenness was occasionally employed as a mitigating circumstance when a person committed acts of violence. Local efforts to disengage behavior while under the influence from dominant cultural sanctions against intratribal violence suggest that at least some community members interpreted drunkenness as a "time out" (MacAndrew and Edgerton 1969) from usual behavioral expectations.

These accounts suggest that in this era drinking was locally interpreted as pathological by some, but this determination was often conditional rather than amounting to a broad call for temperance. Responses to drinking-related problems ranged from tolerance to active intervention, from the disciplinary actions of military societies to the ritual innovations of the chief's society. This heterogeneity of understandings and responses continued in subsequent decades, although shaped in new ways by changing conditions.

Expanding Alcohol Use and Emergent Health Services

By virtually all accounts, the decades between 1930 and 1970 witnessed a significant rise in drinking rates at Northern Cheyenne. Correspondingly, the ambiguity and diversity of meanings associated with alcohol seem to have intensified. Frequent drinking became normalized and even normative in some segments of the community, while other segments continued to identify and decry drinking-related problems in both public and private settings. The latter increasingly drew upon newly emergent discourses about alcohol in non-Native society, including those developed within the Twelve Steps of Alcoholics Anonymous. This era also witnessed the first institutionalized service programs to address alcohol-related problems on the reservation.

While ethnohistorical interviews and published records agree that alcohol use had increased sharply on the reservation by 1950, specific dates vary. Liberty records that alcohol use "did not become serious among the Northern Cheyennes until about 1925. Drinking accelerated in the 1930s when deep discouragement set in following the failure of government programs in cattle raising, dry farming, and relief" (Stands in Timber and Liberty 1998:274f). Yet while Weist affirms that this time period was psychologically difficult for many Cheyennes, he maintains that most did not resort to alcohol: "A few Cheyennes sought to ease their frustrations by drinking; however, most simply endured as best they could" (Weist 1978:18). Hoebel also places the date somewhat later: "The Northern Cheyenne were, until after WWII, looked upon by many outsiders as 'conservative.' It is true that in their isolation, and due to 'benign neglect' by the Bureau of Indian Affairs, they retained much of their identity and sense of self-worth and dignity. The Northern Cheyennes of the 1930s were poor—but proud. There was little alcoholism or serious social despair" (1978:131). Stella (Sunny) Peters, who worked as a nurse on the reservation for over five decades, also observes in her memoir that "the lifestyle of the people included no drug or alcohol abuse" (1992:21) when she first arrived in Lame Deer in 1942.

These discrepancies may well reflect how rising drinking rates took an uneven course, occurring earlier among some families or community sectors and later among others. Most people that I interviewed identified World War II and the subsequent lifting of federal prohibition as seminal events in the rise of alcohol use on the reservation. As Esther, born in the late 1920s, recounted: "In my school years there were certain ones who had parties and drank, but I didn't go to those. Then around World War II, everything went haywire. Those men in the service, they had kind of a hard time over there. Like my husband, I never knew him to drink until he got back. Then Eisenhower passed a bill that enabled Indians to drink in bars." As part of termination-era legislation in the United States, federal laws prohibiting the purchase and consumption of alcohol by Native Americans were repealed in 1952. Individual reservation communities voted on whether or not to maintain prohibition as a tribal law, and the Northern Cheyennes joined the approximately two-thirds of federally recognized tribes who voted to continue it (May 1982).[4]

It is important to clarify that whether federal or tribal, these laws have never fully limited access to alcohol on reservation lands. Several bars are located just over the reservation line, and alcohol can also be purchased in grocery and liquor stores in various off-reservation towns located 20–60 miles from Lame Deer. In addition, local practices of bootlegging have never been uncommon. Law enforcement in a rural area is inherently difficult, and given limited alternatives, alcohol and drug trafficking are some of the most profitable local business ventures available. Instead of restricting use, the clearest effect of prohibition laws has been to occupy much of the caseload of the tribal courts and police with alcohol- and drug-related offenses such as possession, sales, public drunkenness, and driving while intoxicated.

While the shift from federal to tribal prohibition may have indeed enhanced the community's access to alcohol, it seems probable that other local conditions also contributed. These include a greater availability of cash with the influx of New Deal jobs, rising access to cars, and road improvements on the reservation by the 1940s. Sara, born in the 1930s, recalled the infrequency of drinking among community members in her early childhood: "In my time, it was something to see someone drunk. It affected the whole village. I remember this one man would be drunk and driving around, and everyone was out after dark watching him. It wasn't all the time, though. We never had that much money, and nobody really had cars." She explicitly links alcohol use with access to both cash and cars. While all of these factors help to explain access, however, they do not specifically explain why the greater availability of alcohol on the reservation was accompanied by motivation to use it. The statements above by Liberty, Weist, and Hoebel invoke the familiar psychosocial theories of demoralization and frustration, but their accuracy is difficult to assess without detailed information about the personal experiences or motivations of community members who started drinking in this era. By the 1990s, I was able to document only older community members' recollections of witnessing a marked transition in drinking rates circa the 1940s and 1950s.

Sara's description of life in the 1930s contrasts markedly with those of community members born in the 1950s, for example. Louise portrayed alcohol as a near-daily presence in her home life during this decade:

When I was younger, I thought that was just the way of life. I thought that's the way it was. [The kids would be] playing around while they [the adults] are sitting around drinking. And then like next morning they would sit around and talk about what they did yesterday, or what they remembered they did the night before, and if it was funny they'd laugh about it. But they would start in again, start drinking again. And it was there, so we just drank it too.

Louise perceived frequent alcohol consumption as normal and started to drink as a small child.

Yet while the notion that drinking was normal and expected seems to have become increasingly prominent on the reservation in this era, alcohol use also continued to be identified as a problem in public commentary. Records of statements by prominent tribal leaders like John Woodenlegs specifically identify rising levels of drinking as an important threat to personal and collective well-being. The first program founded to address alcohol-related problems on the reservation was established within this climate, during the late 1950s.[5]

Limited records make it difficult to gauge the extent to which the need for this program was identified by Northern Cheyennes themselves, as opposed to federal agencies or others. What is clear is that Northern Cheyenne health services for alcohol reflect broader trends in addiction treatment in the United States, yet also the unique impact of local cultural understandings of alcohol and the peculiar dynamics of political and economic resources for health services on the reservation.

The initial program to address problematic drinking on the reservation was a medical one, consisting of a detoxification ("detox") program run by an Indian Health Service physician. Like other medical treatment programs in this era (White 1998), it relied heavily on prescriptions of disulfiram, which causes a person to become ill if they consume alcohol while it is in their system.

By the 1960s the growing national popularity of halfway houses (White 1998) was also visible at Northern Cheyenne, with the establishment of a residential center where people could stay as they sobered up and prepared to reenter the community. Funding for services improved substantially in this decade, thanks to the Office of Economic Opportunity (part of the federal War on Poverty that aimed to improve living conditions for minorities in the United States) and the founding of the National Institute on Alcohol Abuse and Alcoholism. The Morning Star Recovery Program was founded at Northern Cheyenne in the late 1960s and, like other community-based programs throughout the United States in this era, was based on Twelve Steps of Alcoholics Anonymous.

Interviews with long-time Northern Cheyenne participants in Alcoholics Anonymous (A.A.) suggest that community members first began attending A.A. meetings in significant numbers in the late 1960s and early 1970s. Initially, tribal members attended meetings held off the reservation, such as at the home of a nearby non-Native rancher. Northern Cheyenne men became involved in A.A. first, through church membership and other social ties with non-Native men. Within a few years, some began founding their own groups on the reservation. The first A.A. group specifically for Northern Cheyenne women was organized in the mid-1970s, by women who were attending A.A. with their husbands and finding that the associated Al-Anon meeting, intended for "wives of alcoholics" in original A.A. practice, did not address the realities of their own alcohol use.

From this point forward, the alcohol program continued to evolve, but concepts and practices drawn from Twelve Step therapies have remained a mainstay of its services. A local cultural landscape of ideas, values, and resources has shaped the impact of national trends in addiction therapy on Northern Cheyenne alcohol services and has also linked distinctive local meanings and social consequences with Twelve Step therapies on the reservation.

Normative Substance Use and Professionalized Addiction Services

By the 1970s, evidence mounts that drinking and drug use were normative for increasing segments of the Northern Cheyenne community. Ethnographers Straus and Weist both attest to the widespread significance of drinking in reservation life by circa 1970. Weist (1971) noted that the "drinker/nondrinker" distinction served as one of the most salient dimensions of social identity, besides gender and kinship, that oriented community members' relationships with one another. Straus observed that Northern Cheyenne children were disciplined by reference to a variety of threatening figures, including the new-style "wino," alongside the more traditional Cheyenne bogeyman or méstaa'e (1976:210).

My interviews elicited numerous portraits of substance use as an integral feature of young adulthood by this era. Such associations are certainly not unique to the Cheyennes or other Native Americans (as student behavior on many American college and university campuses amply demonstrates!). Yet local conceptualizations of the life course at

Northern Cheyenne also promote a tendency to normalize substance use among youth. My findings here affirm those of Straus (1976, 1977), who conducted rich ethnopsychological studies at Northern Cheyenne in the 1970s. Straus documented a local conceptualization that four spirits make up a person. Two are "good," and two are "crazy" (1976:163). A person also includes a dimension of knowledge and action. Thus, one can have good spirits that are in control of knowledge (i.e., be very wise) but act in crazy ways (i.e., one's actions are guided by crazy spirits) (1976:165). Crazy behavior contradicts prominent local cultural values and includes lying, stealing, fighting, being sexually aggressive or promiscuous, and drinking (1976:164, 165).

Straus emphasizes that this ethnopsychological framework casts "crazy" behavior as a natural part of being human, as Morris also articulated above, and as especially characteristic of youth. People in more mature phases of life are expected to achieve greater conformity with prominent local understandings of wisdom. My own findings affirm Straus's additional description of how local definitions of maturity are not only age- but also gender-specific. For many people, having more than one or two children generally seems to mark the onset of the more mature phase of adulthood, for example, and women are often held to this standard more strictly than men. After this point, persistent drinking is more likely to strike others as a signifier of one's continued (and now inappropriate) presence in a youthful phase of life.

Yet although community members' criticism of persistent heavy drinking by people in later adulthood was common, a pattern of occasional binges or of moderate drinking did not seem to draw significant censure for either men or women. Instead, many Northern Cheyennes seemed to feel that people drink to forget their problems and to have a good time, and as problems are considerable in daily reservation life, the occasional or even frequent use of alcohol was treated as a fact of life by many. It was also clear to me that drinking has continued to be culturally valued as a source of entertaining stories. When community members are called upon or feel the need to tell such a story, the tales not infrequently involve drinking. During interviews, for example, laughter accompanied stories about how one man managed to escape from police during an arrest, despite being handcuffed for an alcohol-related offense; how one woman fought someone several times her size while drunk; and how another man successfully navigated a local road with hairpin turns at high speed while driving in an alcohol-induced blackout.

Local determinations of what constitutes pathological drinking are oriented by perceptions of not simply whether, but more importantly how, alcohol is used. People commonly observe how some community members use on a daily basis, some limit their use to concentrated weekend doses, some use heavily for an evening every now and again, and still others use moderately. While daily use is more likely to be criticized, there is no clear consensus that any of these patterns is inherently pathological. As Billy (born in the 1960s) elaborated, some local parameters for determining when drinking is problematic have to do with consequences more than use patterns: "The way we were taught, it was all right to use alcohol moderately, but when you start abusing it [then you are] spending all your money on it instead of on your family or your needs, bills and stuff . . . not being responsible when you're using."

For many, the variable qualities of particular substances also play a key role in these reckonings. A hierarchy of intoxicating substances is evident in community members' determinations of what constitutes "problem" drinking. For alcohol itself, beer is considered mildest, with hard liquor and wine suggesting the possibility (though not necessarily signifying) that a person might have a more serious drinking problem. Another order of substances, cheaper and used by some community members when alcohol is not available, included Lysol, hair spray, and rubbing alcohol. For most community members, use of these (particularly on a regular basis) signifies that a person has a more serious problem. A ranking of drugs is also frequently evident in people's accounts of substance use, with marijuana being viewed as the mildest, and methamphetamine (locally termed "crank") as the most indicative of more serious problems.

As such, by many community members' standards, the people with "real" problems with alcohol are visible. These people spend the warm months camping in a hollow near Jimtown (the closest bar, located less than a quarter of a mile from the northern reservation border), who hang around in front of the store in Lame Deer and ask others for money, whose noses are red and swollen or whose skin is marked by the eruptions that develop from a combination of heavy alcohol use and sun exposure, and who (if female) bear children with Fetal Alcohol Effect or Fetal Alcohol Syndrome.

Debate also arises around the issue of whether a person should be held fully responsible for his or her behavior while under the influence. In an echo from earlier eras, some Northern Cheyennes continue to employ drunkenness as a mitigator of responsibility: "I hit her, but I was in a blackout"; "he hit me, but only when he was drunk"; (when confronted with molestation) "I was drunk and did not know what I was doing." The frequency of such claims attests to the continuing vitality of a linkage between drunkenness and a "time out" from usual behavioral expectations in local responses to alcohol.

Yet, as in previous eras too, themes of conditional tolerance and acceptance of alcohol use are neither universally shared nor clearly dominant over alternative perspectives at Northern Cheyenne. Drinking and drug use are frequently highlighted as local problems by community leaders at public events and in policy making, as well as in household discussions of daily events in the lives of family members. As with other community problems, alcohol provokes debate among different sectors of the community. Women were more likely to frame the consequences of men's drinking and violence to be more seriously disruptive than men themselves did, for example, and women of younger generations were also somewhat more likely than those of older generations to voice this perspective.

Services for alcohol-related health problems in recent decades have not explicitly responded to this localized diversity of perspectives or their associated politics. By the 1970s various federal agencies had begun describing alcohol as the "number one health problem" facing Native peoples in the United States. In so doing, many used the term *alcoholism* without clear definition, affirming popular assumptions that all forms of drinking by Native peoples were pathological (May 1994; Quintero 2001). The potential for conflict between such broad conceptualizations of pathology and the local understandings described above is clear. The greater investment of funds in alcohol services by the 1970s also brought increasing pressures toward professionalization, including staff training and certification by external agencies. While Northern Cheyenne is not unique in experiencing such pressures (White 1998), they have combined with limited local economic resources to further impact the capacity of alcohol services to respond to the reservation's local cultural complexities.

With the passage of the Indian Health Care Improvement Act in the mid-1970s, the administration of Native American alcohol programs shifted from the National Institute on Alcohol Abuse and Alcoholism to the Indian Health Service. The Northern Cheyenne tribe received a large federal grant to develop an outpatient program, based again on a halfway house, and to contract for detox services. Program staff members were predominantly paraprofessional, primarily Northern Cheyennes who had achieved sobriety, and the program was run by Tribal Health Services. Federal funding for reservation health care services is channeled through two institutions, Tribal Health Services (locally termed Tribal Health) and the U.S. Public Health Service's Indian Health Service (IHS). Nationwide civil rights activism in the 1960s and 1970s and the passage of the Indian Self-Determination and Education Assistance Act of 1975 have supported greater local control of health services, and from that point forward Tribal Health has taken over the administration of an increasing number of health programs from IHS. The two institutions have a complex relationship, since the former is guided by the elected tribal government and the latter by federal (and oftentimes regional, since the IHS is divided into 12 area offices) priorities. These differences and associated histories of tension between the two complicate local control of health programs by Tribal Health in practice (see chapter 7).

Known as the Alcoholism Project by the mid-1970s, the reservation's alcohol program grew to include considerable community outreach (e.g., staff members would go and talk to people in their homes and at the bars). The Alcoholism Project remained closely tied to local A.A. groups, and referred clients to them. Evaluations of this era are mixed. Some former staff members portray it as something of a golden age, when outreach and follow-up were integral parts of the program and contributed to a high success rate for clients. Yet most stories are dominated by the theme of "the revolving door": People would come in when referred by police or courts, or when they were feeling sick; get checked in; dry out; get some education and perhaps get referred to an inpatient treatment center off the reservation; and then go out and start drinking again.[6] Although some people did achieve lasting sobriety during this time, a number of clients and staff members report they were bothered by the fact that after a while, the clients seemed to be the same small group of people cycling back and forth between sobriety and drinking. The program itself was also characterized by considerable instability, changing locations every two years or so and experiencing a high turnover of staff members.

By the 1980s the foundation of the 1990s–2000s Recovery Center had taken form. Twelve Step approaches remained central, grounded in A.A. but heavily influenced by the rise of Adult Children of Alcoholics (ACOA) and codependency therapies. Its services clearly but only partly reflected broader national trends in addiction treatment. As White (1998) describes, by the early 1990s such trends included more integrated ideas about "substance abuse" and "chemical dependency," which cast problems with alcohol as sharing fundamental similarities with other drugs; and a general rise in consensus that both the causes of addiction and therapies for recovery are multiple. Critics argued against key ideas conventionalized by Twelve Step approaches, such as the notion that abstinence is the only reasonable goal of recovery, and pointed out the need to cultivate a broader range of interventions that are better grounded in clinical and theoretical work in psychology and psychiatry. Advocates of cognitive-behavioral therapies, motivational interviewing, shorter-term "rational recovery" self-help groups that focus on self-efficacy rather than a higher power, and other efforts all provided alternatives to Twelve Step approaches (White 1998), with some explicitly challenging the scientific and clinical efficacy of the latter (Fingarette 1989; Miller 2008; Peele 1989). This era also included heightened concern with better attending to the diversity of substance abuse problems by making clearer distinctions between "abuse" and "dependency"; better gauging the timing of therapeutic interventions through more sophisticated "biopsychosocial" assessments of clients; and utilizing more case management approaches that aimed to connect clients with multiple problems beyond alcohol and/or drug use to helpful resources (e.g., for comorbid mental health problems, domestic violence, child welfare, and other concerns).

At the Northern Cheyenne Recovery Center, expanded definitions of "chemical dependency" were visible in efforts to deal with multiple drug, especially methamphetamine, problems on the reservation. Yet many staff told me that they viewed abuse of different substances as fundamentally different kinds of diseases that were difficult to address with current therapies. Use of biopsychosocial assessment and case management techniques, alongside efforts to improve connections with other mental health and social service resources for clients, were integrated into Recovery Center services. Yet the criticisms of Twelve Step approaches taking place on a national level seem to have had limited impact. Many key staff members made comments to me such as, "The Twelve Steps work. We don't know anything that works better," and Recovery Center services continued to emphasize Twelve Step hallmarks such as overcoming denial that one is an alcoholic and relying on a higher power.

Local resources for training and hiring staff may have contributed to this continuing reliance on the Twelve Steps. A chemical dependency counselor training program instituted at the local tribal college in the

1980s served as the key resource for staff education and heavily emphasized a Twelve Step framework, given the interests and orientation of its founder and key instructor. Moreover, available local mental health professionals who were trained in cognitive-behavioral and other therapies that could provide alternatives to Recovery Center's approaches were hired through the Indian Health Service. While individual exceptions were numerous, Recovery Center's connections with IHS mental health programs were generally not reliable or sustained in this era, but infused with the ongoing tensions between Tribal Health and IHS.

The ways in which Recovery Center's staffing and diagnostic and referral practices had become profoundly centered on Twelve Step approaches by the 1990s are historically situated rather than inevitable. In theory, multiple possibilities for a therapeutic program for addiction were feasible by this era, so long as they could be articulated in ways that met contemporary standards for coherence set by funding and regulatory agencies. First, despite growing national criticism, a strong case could be made for the Twelve Steps as a well-known and widespread form of addiction treatment. Alternative mental health therapies with a reasonable evidence base in non-Native research and clinical experience could also be advocated. Finally, a clearly defined therapeutic program expressly designed for Native Americans (e.g., Coyhis and White 2002) or based on "Cheyenne culture" could be proposed and defended. Despite interest in and awareness of all three, a combination of pressures seems to have produced an ongoing investment in the first of these options in Northern Cheyenne alcohol services through recent decades.

To be able to bill a wider range of federal programs for services, counseling staff at Recovery Center were required to achieve accreditation through the regional Northwest Indian Council on Chemical Dependency in the 1980s, and by the more stringent standards of a state chemical dependency certification program by the mid-1990s. Recovery Center's program itself also earned accreditation through the Committee on Accreditation of Rehabilitation Facilities (CARF). As one health administrator clarifies: "What CARF lets you do is, any kind of treatment that is acceptable to them or anywhere else just has to be written down. And you just have to follow your procedures, you've got to document that. For example, you could actually incorporate Cheyenne cultural stuff into their program." Indeed, one major effort to improve the cultural appropriateness of Recovery Center's services has involved the development of a "Traditional Component." My findings document that as of 2005 this program had been initiated and discussed for over a decade, but not fully implemented as an institutionalized resource for Recovery Center's clients or incorporated into its services. Many Recovery Center staff see conflicts in some of its proposed strategies, such as referring clients to traditional spiritual activities. Questions about whether specialists in such activities have or support sobriety are central here, since having high degrees of knowledge about and involvement in these activities is no guarantee of any particular attitude toward sobriety.

One long-time counselor describes additional problems: "We want to incorporate traditional ways into the program, but some traditional people recommend going right to carrying a pipe[7] and making that kind of commitment. I don't want to start there, that is too intense—because if you make a commitment with a pipe and don't follow through, you're going to hurt somebody. Hurt you, or some family member, or some extended family member." For him, the self-transformation of sobriety often has too nebulous and unclear a course to be connected to such high-order ritual activities. Here too we see how orienting services around "tradition" can engage local controversies that have emerged on the reservation stemming from a conflict between beliefs that spiritual power is dangerous unless engaged by people with the appropriate levels of specialized knowledge, and the rising involvement in Cheyenne ritual life of groups whose participation has historically been limited (e.g., women of childbearing age, tribal members who do not speak Cheyenne, and so forth). Given these complexities, formulating clear and coherent definitions of "Cheyenne culture" to be used in addiction treatment is fraught with difficulty and controversy.

Recovery Center's central functions are to provide outpatient services and referrals to inpatient treatment centers. Clients are routed through an initial evaluation for chemical dependency, and local services include one-to-one counseling sessions, prevention education classes, and a six-week intensive outpatient therapy group. Evidence of more severe problems results in referral to residential treatment centers located in a variety of sites across the northern Plains and Pacific Northwest. Recovery Center's diagnostic procedures and program content are based on a combination of psychiatric criteria (from the fourth edition of the *Diagnostic and Statistical Manual of Mental Disorders* [American Psychiatric Association 1994]), American Society of Addiction Medicine standards, and most centrally, Twelve Step approaches. A.A. and related Twelve Step groups (Al-Anon, ACOA, and CoDA, for example) continue on the reservation and surrounding areas. A flyer available at Recovery Center in the summer of 2005 listed 22 such meetings within a 60-mile radius of Lame Deer. Recovery Center services are available free to enrolled tribal members. Most clients are referred through the tribal courts, probation, and social service systems, as these are the prominent local institutions likely to encounter alcohol-related legal and social problems. Some clients arrive through pressure from family members, however, and a small minority also seek out help on their own.

Since the 1980s Recovery Center services have especially incorporated elements from ACOA and codependency therapies, and concepts of historical trauma from national movements specific to Native American mental health. While guided by these nonlocal approaches, Recovery Center staff do make efforts to better adapt their institutional practices to local needs. Counseling staff especially recognize the limitations of Twelve Step approaches. Some modify key Twelve Step concepts and practices in their efforts to help clients, or work to accommodate local interest in using Cheyenne spiritual traditions to support sobriety. Yet through 2005 no systematic efforts to address local needs had been clearly or consistently institutionalized, beyond efforts to better facilitate understanding of Twelve Step concepts among reservation residents. Local critiques of Recovery Center are widespread and reflect the ways in which the local diversity in understandings of alcohol have generated multiple pathways toward sobriety.

Pluralism in Sobriety

Efforts to define and address alcohol-related problems on the Northern Cheyenne Reservation reflect the wider-ranging rhetorical politics visible in commentary about other contemporary community problems. For example, some Northern Cheyennes cast alcohol as less of a threat than other dimensions of colonization, such as increasing loss of language or disruptions in kinship structures. Others position alcohol as a primary cause of these and other problems. Still others prioritize declining knowledge of ritual protocol as a central cause of all collective troubles.

These perspectives can charter quite different paths toward sobriety. Some Northern Cheyennes say that they "quit on their own," without specifying any particular resources used. Others describe a range of resources that helped them to get and to stay sober, including religious institutions (local evangelical Christian churches offer important support for sobriety among their followers) and local ritual activities, nondrinking social activities, and institutionalized services available through Recovery Center. Examples of conflicting responses to Recovery Center's services illustrate some of the key politics of how these different approaches to sobriety interact in local social life.

Many clients and community members on the reservation dispute the accuracy of key terms and definitions commonly used at Recovery Center. The routine use of diagnostic labels of "dependency" or "abuse" clearly conflict with locally prevalent understandings of alcohol-related pathology. Several community members commented to me that everyone who goes into Recovery Center gets labeled as having an illness or a problem, yet when participating in group meetings there, they perceived profound differences between participants. For them, the credibility of the overall program was undermined by the inability of its diagnostic categories to capture what they themselves saw as important distinctions between forms of drinking that seriously undermine one's ability to fulfill one's social responsibilities and those that primarily enact locally accepted social or developmental roles (e.g., youthful risk taking).

Medical anthropologists document similar instances of how tension and debate emerge in numerous cultural contexts when conflicts arise between local understandings of health problems and the diagnostic categories that institutionalized medical services provide for health conditions ranging from infertility (Inhorn 1994) to diabetes (Smith-Morris 2005) to mental illness (Kohrt and Harper 2008). At Northern Cheyenne, the markedly different perspectives on Twelve Step therapies that Louise and Morris articulate are echoed widely throughout the Northern Cheyenne community and can produce social tension.

On yet another social occasion, for example, Morris came away from a conversation with a relative in recovery and commented to me with some irritation that he didn't think that her sobriety made her better than someone who occasionally drank, like himself. "Sometimes I get a little bit crazy," he concluded. While Twelve Step adherents would tend to dismiss such statements as evidence of "denial," this comment also indexes distinctive local ethnopsychological understandings of personal behavior and its control. As mentioned above, "crazy" actions are often not categorically condemned so much as considered to be part of the human condition, and many community members appreciate the entertainment value of telling stories about such actions. To honor this perspective requires one to focus on the good in a person, rather than expressing undue surprise or criticism at imperfections. Morris's response to his relative highlights the power plays that may result when these more flexible local understandings of occasional "crazy" interludes are pathologized by a Twelve Step focus on permanent abstinence. As noted above, many community members indicate that they do not see alcoholism as a condition or disease that relates to the specific amounts or frequencies of one's drinking, for example, and find drinking to be acceptable so long as it does not unduly interfere with one's gender- and age-specific responsibilities (e.g., providing for one's family, caring for children, completing one's schooling, and so forth) (see also O'Nell and Mitchell 1996).

Many also convey special dislike for adopting the label of "alcoholic" or "chemically dependent" while expressing themselves in Recovery Center activities (see also Spicer 2001). While negative reactions to these labels and other conventionalized styles of Twelve Step self-expression are not unique to Northern Cheyennes or other Native American groups (Madsen 1974), they seem to be intensified by local cultural understandings of the power of language to constitute reality (a widespread language ideology documented by ethnographers in numerous cultural contexts). Within the health care system, for instance, Northern Cheyenne staff and patients were sometimes deeply offended by negative prognostic statements by physicians, such as, "I don't think he'll make it through the night." Such statements tempt fate and disrespect the other-than-human powers at work in determining a person's survival. From this perspective, adopting a label such as "alcoholic" promotes an identity that actually impedes rather than facilitates a process of self-transformation in sobriety.

Special concerns about present and future disenfranchisement also underwrite some clients' discomfort with Recovery Center. Several expressed concern about how the inclusion of "chemical dependency" or other diagnostic labels in their medical record might affect their future eligibility for employment, health insurance, or military service.

A number of Northern Cheyennes also question whether a person has the social authority to offer advice to others simply by virtue of their educational credentials and place of work, finding encouragement for behavior change to be most acceptable when it comes from someone who knows them well and who clearly demonstrates a sense of caring and respect for their well-being. Many elaborate that such a person would ideally have established a respectable standing in the community by founding a household, supporting a family, and living in accordance with values of generosity, intergenerational respect, and other local signifiers of maturity and well-being. In a small community, details of the personal lives of Recovery Center staff members are often widely known, and critics especially emphasize instances of current marital or family discord in comments that question the institutional basis for staff members' authority. Many of these comments reflect the broader local rhetorical conventions that surround claims about cultural identity, evaluating staff members in terms of how "really" Cheyenne they are.

In addition to articulating such local ethnopsychologies and modes of evaluating social authority, criticism of Recovery Center highlights local alternatives to institutionalized health services for transforming drinking behavior within the community. Joe is a charismatic administrator in health and social service programs on the reservation, and an often vocal critic of Recovery Center. In one conversation he offered a particularly striking allegorical story about the role of community support in sobriety, describing how he encouraged a man with a drinking problem to bless the food at a public event, introducing him and praising his family. The man was caught off guard and embarrassed by his dirty clothes, but Joe accompanied him and stood by him while he did so. Motivated and energized by this experience, the man went on to sober up and go back to school.

Whatever the factual basis of this story, Joe clearly communicates an alternative to Recovery Center's approaches to supporting sobriety. His comments frame drinking as a problem whose resolution requires reorienting one's experience of self, but he specifies how engaging in locally esteemed activities (such as leading prayer) can help. Rather than institutionalized psychological therapies, Joe's story places acts of generosity and support from others in the community as central motivations for positive transformations in a person's behavior. It calls for collective moral responsibility for others' behavior, and poses fundamental questions about the possibility and desirability of allocating these responsibilities to an institutionalized health program.

These comments by Recovery Center clients and other community members document the vitality of alternatives to Twelve Step approaches to defining alcohol-related problems, as well as for representing self and self-transformation in sobriety, on the Northern Cheyenne Reservation. For proponents of Recovery Center's Twelve Step approach, substance use and addiction overlap tightly. Sobriety entails a self-conscious process of psychological transformation that is motivated by an intense desire to change and evidenced by the learning of new terms, engaging a more reflexive mode of experience, new self-representational practices (e.g., as "alcoholic"), and the expressive release of emotions. Proponents also view the professional credentials of staff members as at least partially legitimate. Critics, however, engage alternative local ethnopsychological constructions of self and emotion in relation to substance use and posit quite different foundations for legitimate social authority. For example, expressions of generosity and caring, as indexed by Joe's allegorical story above, carry far greater weight with some community members than professional credentials and titles. Critics also voiced suspicions about other institutional practices at Recovery Center that clearly derive from Anglo-American norms, from pedagogical practices to medico-legal surveillance.

Many Northern Cheyennes simply do not view drinking and drunkenness as inherently or universally problematic. While ethnohistorical and ethnographic sources record a long history of negative responses to drinking and its consequences, they also document a long legacy of viewing both alcohol consumption and drunken behavior as benign and/or entertaining. My findings indicate that both of these interpretations intensified in community discourse after World War II, when local drinking rates rose sharply. Community members at Northern Cheyenne continue to offer a spectrum of different answers to the questions of how alcohol figures among threats to Cheyenne well-being, as well as what sobriety entails.

Northern Cheyennes who want to stop drinking frequently do not seek out help from Recovery Center but work to quit on their own. Their strategies are largely centered on avoiding their drinking buddies and cultivating other sources of meaning and purpose in life. These therapeutic elements are also shared by Twelve Step approaches, but "quitting on one's own" includes tapping into a somewhat different set of resources. Key strategies involve developing new social activities and a new social circle through activities like joining a women's beadwork group or visiting more with kin who do not drink. Also prominent among these strategies are engaging in local spiritual practices such as sweat lodge, fasting, and Sun Dance. Again, only a limited number of participants in these practices are seeking sobriety, however (see also Medicine 2007), and people involved in Recovery Center also employ these practices. As such, spiritual practices serve as a common cultural arena for community members who have diverse goals and motivations, but who share a general investment in ritual practice as a response to pressing personal or collective problems. Yet entering into the arena of spiritual practices involves encountering the controversies that accompany it.

A closer examination of the experiences and accounts of Northern Cheyenne community members' personal experiences with drinking and sobriety helps to illustrate these complexities, to describe how and for whom Twelve Step approaches hold the most appeal on the reservation, and to offer a richer discussion of some of the intertwining psychological and sociopolitical reasons for this selective appeal. This analysis also highlights how even proponents of Twelve Step approaches on the reservation express criticism of some of their elements and work to modify them to better fit local realities. Efforts by younger generations of women to couple Twelve Step approaches with new degrees and forms of participation in local ritual practices, for example, especially have sparked a complex mixture of support and criticism from the Northern Cheyenne community. While criticism of Twelve Step approaches certainly occurs in other communities, the constellation of criticisms, their rhetorical forms, and their social consequences at Northern Cheyenne bear a distinctly local sensibility. Much support for sobriety on the reservation is taking place at a grassroots level, and prominently includes some women's efforts to modify Twelve Step approaches for local use. The next three chapters examine what women's accounts reveal about how gender and generation can shape subjective experience, perception, and action with regard to alcohol-related health problems on the reservation.

Part II
Women's Narratives
Social Positioning, Subjectivity, and Sobriety

While Twelve Step approaches lack generalized appeal at Northern Cheyenne, they are engaged by some community members in their efforts toward sobriety, most notably by women of younger generations. When I first asked why, many community members suggested that younger women were more motivated by their roles as caregivers to children, and that the styles of open emotional expression encouraged by the Twelve Steps were more consonant with local cultural expectations of women than of men. My initial research affirmed the importance of gender in shaping social roles and the cultural patterning of emotional expression, but it also raised additional questions. For example, I soon noticed clear generational differences among women, in addition to the gender differences between women and men. Moreover, many younger women clearly made selective and creative use of Twelve Step concepts (e.g., alcoholism) and departed from its conventional practices (e.g., regularly attending meetings).

To better understand local patterns in the appeal and use of the Twelve Steps on the reservation, I interviewed an array of Northern Cheyenne women about their life histories, with a special focus on experiences with drinking and sobriety. All were women who described drinking as problematic, positioning alcohol as a significant threat to well-being in their personal, family, and/or community's lives. Almost all had also engaged in a pattern of heavy, frequent drinking at some point in their lives, and had later either quit drinking entirely or significantly reduced their use of alcohol.

Patterned differences in form and content distinguished the narratives of women born before and after approximately 1950. Women of older generations described growing up in a coherent world in which social relationships were grounded in collaboration and respect, and then witnessing emergent drinking and violence erode this world. An idiom of "forgetting" dominated their accounts of these changes.

In contrast, women of younger generations portrayed growing up when drinking and violence had become widespread, and described social relationships in their early lives significantly in terms of abuse and neglect. Their accounts emphasized a conceptualization of "cycles" that figures prominently in ACOA- and codependency-oriented Twelve Step therapies, in which painful experiences are reproduced over time until healed through recovery. These distinct ways of talking about drinking and sobriety reflect patterned differences in how Northern Cheyenne women born before and after 1950 variously employ, challenge, and modify the prominent rhetorical conventions evident in local commentary about community problems on the reservation. They stem in part from how distinctive subjectivities or modes of feeling, interpretation, and action have emerged from different generations' experiences and help to explain the selective appeal of different therapeutic resources for sobriety to women from different generational groups.

Generation and gender also figure in the community members' responses to women who become sober or who publicly advocate for sobriety. While reflecting the general dynamics of local commentary about community problems, these responses also highlight the specific politics associated with changing gender roles and relations on the reservation. For the first time in recorded reservation history, the generation of Northern Cheyenne women born in the early 1970s have a higher employment rate than do Northern Cheyenne men (Ward and Wilson 1989). By the 1980s and 1990s, Northern Cheyenne women were also moving into a number of higher administrative positions in social and educational programs. Women's representation in the Tribal Council increased by these years, and both postmenopausal and younger women started to play visibly active roles in spiritual practices—fasting in the hills, in the Sun Dance lodge, or at Bear Butte; attending and sometimes running their own sweat lodges; and participating more vocally in various decision-making forums regarding the Sun Dance, Sacred Buffalo Hat, and other local ritual practices.

These changes have frequently met with controversy. Women's participation in ceremonial life is vigorously criticized by some men. Though women's employment seems to have remained fairly stable during the last 15 years, representation on the Tribal Council underwent a dramatic shift. In 1994 the Tribal Council was 25–30 percent female, but after community elections in 1996, 1998, and 2000, it again became over 90 percent male. Subsequent election years have favored more female candidates once again. The year 2000 also witnessed the election of the first Northern Cheyenne woman to the position of tribal president, yet her four-year term in office provoked intense debate. A set of male Tribal Council members especially challenged her authority, for example by organizing collective no-shows at a number of council meetings, such that a quorum could not be reached and tribal business could not be completed.

The next three chapters compare and contrast the form and content of personal narratives produced by women born before and after 1950, to illuminate how gender and generation intersect to produce patterns in both subjective experience (i.e., perception, thought, feeling, motivation) and styles of talking. I argue here that midcentury changes in reservation life have positioned generations differently in relation to broader local cultural constructions of development, personhood, and gender, and have produced patterned differences in personal experience that are both psychologically and socially significant for individual women.

Constructing two broad generational categories is clearly an analytic convenience that tends to downplay the diversity within each group in order to foreground differences between the two. As will become clear, the conditions experienced on a widespread basis by "younger" women were not universal among women born after 1950, appearing earlier in select households and families to affect some "older" women. Similarly, not all older women feel alienated from Twelve Step approaches, and by no means do all younger women on the reservation feel attracted to them. With these complexities in mind, each chapter includes excerpts from a number of women's narratives to consider the individual diversity evident in their accounts as well as broader patterns of difference.

Given how these life history narratives focus on experiences of threatened well-being, I consider them to be forms of "illness narratives," or stories that concern experiences of suffering and efforts toward their therapeutic resolution. Anthropologists frequently define illness narratives as stories that emplot coherence, and analyze how such stories reflect their tellers' efforts to ameliorate the disruptive effects of experiences that violate what is desired, expected, and otherwise intelligible within their local moral world (Becker 1997; Kleinman 1988). These works describe how narrative facilitates the restoration of a self disoriented by suffering.[1] Narrative analysis also has a rich history in medical, psychological, and feminist anthropology as a tool for illuminating subjective experience (Langness and Frank 1981; Mattingly and Garro 2000; Personal Narratives Group 1989).

Narrative Analysis and the Cultural Politics of Persuasion

Anthropologists are increasingly exploring the political contexts for expressions and representations of subjective experiences of suffering (Kleinman et al. 1997). As storytellers, narrators work to fashion a persuasive account not only for themselves, but also for socially significant others (Mattingly and Garro 2000). Narrative emplotment figures as one of a number of discursive tools in the aftermath of state-sponsored acts of violence, for instance, utilized by survivors in their claims for recognition and restitution (Zarowsky 2004). Yet the implications of narratives of suffering for immediate social relationships within localized communities, while certainly recognized (Good and Good 1994), remain relatively unexplored in recent ethnographic works, which tend to focus on other important discursive arenas, such as international media coverage (Kleinman and Kleinman 1997), specialized state legal venues (Ross 2001), or the local institutional contexts of clinics and hospitals (Kirmayer 2000; Mattingly 1998). Notable exceptions include Hunt (2000), who analyzes illness narratives among Latinas with cancer as efforts not only to imbue coherence in their experiences of suffering, but also to transform troubling interpersonal relationships. Similarly, O'Nell analyzes how Native American veterans on the northern Plains shift genres in telling their war stories, arguing that "psychological talk, like all talk, is both representational [i.e., reflecting experience] and pragmatic [i.e., exerting social consequences]" (2000:442). Both highlight how narratives about sickness and suffering emerge within localized social contexts and can work to transform a teller's social status and/or interpersonal relationships.

Strategies of persuasion are particularly salient for individuals pursuing sobriety at Northern Cheyenne. Social pressures to drink can be intense for both youth and adults, as in other northern Plains reservation communities where drinking is prevalent (e.g., Bezdek and Spicer 2006). Reducing or quitting drinking therefore involves fashioning and voicing persuasive accounts in support of one's new identity as a nondrinker. These persuasive strategies are discernible in the narratives that speakers produce in ethnographic interviews.

Clearly, the context of an ethnographic interview imposes its own genres of speech, however, shaping the narratives produced. These issues have sparked lively debate in anthropology in recent decades, especially with regard to life history interviews.

Life Histories: Critical Perspectives

Gathering and publishing the life histories of selected individuals was a central task in the early decades of American anthropology, especially relevant to psychological anthropology's efforts to situate individuals within their cultural contexts (Langness and Frank 1981). But by the later decades of the twentieth century, numerous scholars criticized how life histories were too often presented as clear recordings of data for anthropological analysis, obscuring the messier reality of how these accounts actually emerged from interactions between their tellers and the ethnographer (Crapanzano 1980), and were often clearly shaped by the agendas of their tellers (Behar 2003). Linguistic anthropologists especially highlighted the power differentials between researchers and subjects that shape ethnographic interviewing (Briggs 1986), and how these were obscured in the production of published ethnographies. Postcolonial scholars have specifically criticized the life history genre as a "modernist fantasy about society and selfhood" (Comaroff and Comaroff 1992:26) that can impose the subject positions and forms of speech familiar to anthropologists and their audiences, rather than eliciting those of local cultural worlds. These critiques emerged as part of the broader questioning of anthropological knowledge production in the 1980s with the growing influence of poststructuralist theories (Clifford and Marcus 1986), which helped to pose new questions about the nature of ethnography and the need for anthropologists to consider questions of power inherent in their own work (Asad 1995; Deloria 1988) and the lives of those they study.

In response to these serious concerns, one might be tempted to avoid gathering or analyzing life histories altogether. But an alternative to such dismissal is to first consider whether this speech genre is indeed purely imposed by the ethnographer. Are there local practices of personal history telling in a given community? The telling of personal experiences and developmental changes over time can offer ethnographers important insights into local understandings of the life cycle and discourses of self-representation, as well as rich information about subjective perception and experience. For example, Straus (1977) has documented prominent local ethnopsychological constructions of four stages of the life cycle at Northern Cheyenne. The practices of elders who teach by talking, and younger tribal members who learn by listening, form an essential part of this local construction of the life course. Indeed, during my own fieldwork I witnessed numerous instances of personal history telling by elders in the community. Whether humorous or poignant or aiming to convey a particular type of knowledge, all were intended to instruct younger members of the community in proper behavior and responses to life's challenges. Mapping out social patterns and historical changes in who tells such stories and how they tell them can help to illuminate the workings of local structures of power and the debates that surround them.

Conducting interviews in the context of ongoing participant observation can also enrich understanding of such local politics. For example, I recurrently noticed how women's comments referenced alternative viewpoints in their community, both explicitly and implicitly. Attending to this indirect conversation helped me to better understand some of the more public forms of discussion and debate about sobriety, gender, and social authority. Without engaging in pretenses of objectivity, therefore, it seems important to view speech acts like the personal narratives produced in interviews as multidimensional, dealing with immediate but also imagined or habitual audiences.

Several well-known ethnographies also demonstrate how anthropologists can effectively portray how interviewer and interviewee interact during the gathering of life histories (e.g., Behar 2003; Crapanzano 1980) and consider how such encounters are shaped by local standards for interaction with the social groups that interviewers are perceived to embody. In both explicit and subtle ways, Northern Cheyenne women communicated how their varied perceptions of my ethnic, class, and personal background shaped their understandings of our interactions.

Ethnographic Interviewing on the Rez

I became acquainted with most of the women I interviewed through my work in various community settings (e.g., the elderly housing center, tribal college, tribal health outreach programs, and Recovery Center), as well as through the more informal social networks that I had established by my second year of fieldwork. In 1996 I also interviewed a selection of women as part of a joint project with Carol Ward, a sociologist from Brigham Young University who conducted research about recovery for her ongoing work about education and economic development at Northern Cheyenne (Baird-Olson and Ward 2000; Ward 2005). Because of my own conscious efforts to seek out new voices, however, the majority of women I interviewed had little if any prior experience participating in any type of research.

While the women that I interviewed often were connected to one or two others through kinship, employment, neighborhood of residence, or other social ties, I expressly aimed to talk with members of a range of different social groupings on the reservation. I did not, for example, interview mothers and daughters (though doing so would likely offer new layers of psychosocial information about the intergenerational politics that I describe here).

White, female, and in my twenties at the time, I was younger than the majority of women I interviewed and seemingly often elicited a locally conventional instructional mode of speech appropriate when interacting with juniors in the life course. I was sometimes also viewed as a sympathetic person who had already demonstrated her ability to maintain confidentiality among many of the women whom I interviewed. In this way I was structurally akin to a counselor, so some women made use of the interview as a chance to talk at some length about difficulties they had experienced or were currently having in their lives.

Broader local assumptions about non-Natives were clearly visible in how women sometimes assumed that there was a greater gap between my experiences and theirs (one woman asked if I had ever tasted alcohol), or in some cases a greater similarity (one woman clearly but erroneously presumed that I shared her high level of knowledge about Christianity), than in fact existed. Some women explicitly reflected upon previous encounters with non-Natives, constructing a metanarrative about the experience of being interviewed. Most poignantly, one older-generation woman described a childhood opportunity that she'd had to be adopted by a non-Native household. She ended the story by saying that if that had happened, "maybe I wouldn't be here now" being interviewed for a study about alcohol—a comment that expressed an acute awareness of how she was being positioned as a "Northern Cheyenne woman with a history of drinking" in the interview, as well as her own consciousness of unrealized alternatives to her actual life course.

My position as a non-Native clearly shaped interactions during the interviews in other ways too. A few women expressed concern about whether they were providing the "right" answers to my questions, needing reassurance that my purpose was to understand their perceptions and experiences rather than evaluate them in such terms. These concerns are not uncommon in research based on open-ended interviews, but at Northern Cheyenne they may also reflect long histories of unequal power relations and recurrent experiences of being deemed "wrong" for differing from the norms enacted by non-Native institutions.

In these ways women's own interests, perspectives, and priorities clearly shaped the accounts produced in the interviews that I recount here. A number of women explicitly exercised an editorial hand in our encounters, such as regulating how I recorded their speech. In taped interviews, some shared more after the tape recorder was turned off— often about the more outrageous and embarrassing things that they had done in their drinking days. In interviews where I took written notes, women would occasionally tell me, "Don't write this down, but . . . ," and proceed to make comments about their attitudes toward other minority ethnic groups or their religious beliefs and concerns. Also, Northern Cheyenne is a small community, so I often heard stories about women whom I had interviewed, from their family members, neighbors, and so forth, in ways that made visible some of their editing processes in the interviews. For example, I heard from a trusted friend that one woman had been sexually abused by her father as a teenager, either in the sense of being molested by him directly and/or in the sense that he engineered her sexual involvement with other men. The woman had not mentioned anything about this when I interviewed her, and although she did respond to questions about the problem of sexual abuse in the community, she did not do so with any reference to her father. If anything, she presented herself to me in the interviews as having limited experience with men. I did not know this woman especially well but did socialize with her and know that she made comments to others that I was consistently unresponsive to various community members' efforts to engage me in local sexual politics (see chapter 1). She was also aware that I was slightly acquainted with her father through my participation in community activities. These perceptions of me may well have shaped her self-presentation in our encounter.

Subjectivity: Anthropological Perspectives

By gathering and analyzing personal narratives as forms of talk that do not transparently reflect but nonetheless bear some relationship to the speaker's experience, this project also contributes to ongoing discussions in anthropology about how to understand the emergence and experience of subjectivity. In anthropology, the concept of subjectivity most often refers to the processes of feeling, interpretation, and imagination that both shape and are shaped by social experience. For many, not only cultural contexts but also human capacities for self-awareness and embodied experience influence how subjective experiences like thought, emotion, moral evaluation, and motivation are experienced and expressed. In studying these phenomena, some rely on individual accounts to illuminate broader cultural terms and social patterns (e.g., Brodwin 2003), while others employ more person-centered methods that focus on the lived body-self of individuals and more detailed accounts of their thoughts, feelings, and responses to specific situations (e.g., Parish 2008). Yet, while some anthropologists debate the respective merits of these approaches, many treat both as useful in the broader aim of better grasping how subjectivity is formed and renegotiated through a convergence of historical conditions, cultural contexts, and lived experiences of events (e.g., Bacigalupo 2007).

This approach recognizes that an essential feature of human existence is an unpredictable flow of experience that is encountered by individuals, who creatively and selectively make use of available cultural resources as they respond. Its proponents point out that the heavy emphasis on the power politics of talk (discourse) and attention to social positioning in hierarchies that is prioritized in much contemporary social theory can overlook the complex realities of how thoughts and feelings emerge and change through experience and social interaction (B. Good et al. 2008; Linger 1994). As such, while direct access to the "inner" lives of others may not be as straightforward or possible as previous generations of psychological anthropologists tended to assume (Lindholm 2007), subjective experience remains an essential dimension of how human lives are actually lived. Recent formulations of discourse analysis (Brenneis 2000), practice theory (Holland and Leander 2004; Ortner 2006), and postcolonial theory (Good et al. 2008), demonstrate that it is possible for anthropologists to make use of current theoretical and methodological insights while retaining a multifaceted view of human experience and motivation and avoiding the pitfalls of unduly reducing human beings to "social actors" who occupy "subject positions" that generate motives solely oriented around enacting or challenging power relations. In the chapters that follow, I aim to demonstrate how lived experiences, ranging from those in childhood to present-day social interactions, shape Northern Cheyenne women's perceptions and interpretations of alcohol-related problems, influence the ways in which they talk about these issues, and help to account for both their motivations and resources for changing drinking behavior.

The next three chapters highlight key similarities and differences in experiences and representations of alcohol in "older" and "younger" Northern Cheyenne women's life history narratives. The personal narratives presented here were primarily gathered in 1996 and 1997. After first completing a small project of 20 interviews with staff and clients at Recovery Center, including both men and women, I developed a broader, community-based sample of women, completing in-depth interviews with a total of 35 women who self-identified as either being sober or pursuing sobriety. I was able to provisionally confirm women's self-reports of abstaining or significantly restricting their drinking by attending to news and conversation in daily community life, which frequently featured reports (of imperfect but often surprising accuracy, as my closer inquiries revealed) about who was drinking. The women ranged in age from 18 to 84, with the majority in their forties and fifties. Reflecting the general population pattern of the reservation, most of the women were from the most populous district of Lame Deer, with Ashland and Busby following, and then Muddy and Birney.

I have assigned pseudonyms to all of the women interviewed; I have occasionally also assigned multiple names to excerpts from the narrative of a single person, and/or changed minor personal details (about where they are employed, family composition, and so forth). Finally, I have tried to preserve something of the quality of speech on the reservation, including details such as the ways in which past and present verb tenses are sometimes used interchangeably in English spoken by native Cheyenne speakers, and the ways in which people quote the speech of others in telling stories. In a reflection of the decline of Cheyenne language over this century, the majority of women born before 1950 spoke Cheyenne as their first language, while women born in the 1950s were equally divided among Cheyenne and English speakers. Women born in the 1960s and later most often spoke English exclusively, and although many had some understanding of Cheyenne, none spoke it fluently. Given that all women's skills with English were better than my skills with Cheyenne, the interviews were primarily conducted in English, although women fluent in Cheyenne would sometimes move between the two (and either immediately offer a translation or ask me to produce one, which they then affirmed or corrected).

Chapter 4 considers how women's narratives reference prominent local ethnopsychological understandings of the development of Cheyenne personhood and specifically examines how, given their different historical experiences, older and younger women situate alcohol's impact on this process in strikingly different ways. Chapter 5 examines women's descriptions and interpretations of their lives as adults. Older and younger women characterize gender-specific concerns such as forming households and caring for children similarly but also offer distinct explanations for how alcohol has impacted these responsibilities.

Chapter 6 then considers women's narratives of sobriety, pulling these themes together to demonstrate the diverse understandings of sobriety that Northern Cheyenne women have and the very different pathways through which they seek it. This chapter also examines the politics that have accompanied some younger women's public advocacy for sobriety, situating the stories that they tell and actions that they take within the local rhetorical conventions, diversity of perspectives on alcohol, and politics of cultural identity and social authority discussed throughout the preceding chapters. Younger women both use and attempt to transform locally prominent rhetorical conventions as they describe personal and community problems with alcohol, and their advocacy for sobriety therefore engages ongoing community debates about not only changing gender roles and relations, but also cultural identity, the nature of "tradition," and what constitutes legitimate grounds for social authority.

4
Becoming a Person

When Northern Cheyenne women who are concerned about sobriety recount their life histories, alcohol serves as a pervasive referent. Closely attending to their narratives offers insight into how individuals variously engage the numerous rhetorical tools available to them. Women's accounts of childhood and coming of age reveal the different ways in which they position alcohol's impact upon their own development and that of others in the community. For older women, alcohol often figures in a broader process of moral erosion, and their narratives center on themes of how Northern Cheyenne community members have fundamentally changed since their early childhood. Their accounts reflect the rhetorical legacies of Sweet Medicine's prophecies, which emphasize themes of loss in cultural change and the forgetting of past teachings. Younger women, in contrast, position alcohol as a direct cause of disrupted personal development, often drawing much more heavily upon terms and concepts from A.A., ACOA, and codependency therapies. Comparing and contrasting the two generational groups illuminates the complex interplay between local rhetorical conventions and those of the Twelve Steps and suggests that the latter may hold special appeal for community members whose achievement of personhood (in the sense of meeting local cultural understandings of what it means to be human, and standards for functioning as a community member) is compromised within prominent local discourses about becoming and being Northern Cheyenne.

These rhetorical features of women's accounts in part express their current social experiences and agendas, such as seeking sources of discursive authority to legitimate their commentary about alcohol-related problems on the reservation. Yet they also in part seem to reflect how the lived experiences of different generations on the reservation as children and young adults coming of age have been shaped by distinct historical conditions. As such, their rhetorical practices offer insight into both current sociopolitical concerns and psychological efforts to imbue meaning in often difficult and painful experiences.

Older Women's Narratives: Drinking and Moral Erosion

Predominant themes in older women's narratives emphasize how proper social relationships between generations and genders, and proper ritual relationships between humans and the other-than-human powers that populate the Cheyenne world, initially produced a coherent moral world in their early lives. Key to perpetuating this world is the reproduction of core dimensions of local personhood: proper affect and comportment of individuals, and motivation by ethics of generosity and reciprocity, underwrite Cheyenne capacities to engage in smooth relationships and abide by ritual protocol. Older Northern Cheyenne women describe how these capacities began to erode by their young adulthood, and although alcohol clearly figures in their initial comments about this process, they situate drinking among multiple factors that deeply threaten Northern Cheyenne well-being.

Early Childhood: Coherent Moral Worlds

I started all of the life history interviews with a broad question about early childhood memories. Almost universally, older women began with statements that reflect a moral ordering of genders and generations: men served as effective providers, while women acted as stable keepers of homes, and adults watched and taught children, while children listened to adults. While noting how their lives were influenced by non-Native institutions such as churches and schools, for the most part older women's accounts rhetorically contained these to portray reservation life in their childhoods as embedded within an alien world, but not severely disrupted by it.

For example, Vicky's account of growing up in Birney, a small community located just across the reservation border from a non-Native town of the same name, includes central themes of family-centered collaboration and the smooth integration of the Cheyenne and non-Native worlds:

> My dad always held down a job. And he used to plant—hay, alfalfa. Same with my grandpa, he used to plant, and keep chickens, geese, tur- keys. They had a lot of horses, too. My mom used to bead—buckskin

dresses, cradleboards, moccasins, leggings, men's war dance collars. People would ask her to make these things. My aunt and my mom used to teach all us kids how to bead, my cousins too. I really enjoyed that, learning that. My mom was involved in a beading project in Lame Deer—coin purses, eyeglasses, wristbands. Me and my cousin did the edgework on them. I used to hang around with my cousin. We would go walk, hike around Birney, exploring. In the summertime we would fish. We would ride horses a lot, too. There was hardly anything going on. There was a dance hall in white Birney, and they used to have dances there. But it burned down and was never rebuilt. They had Indian dances in Lame Deer and at Rosebud, too. We used to go. Sometimes come to movies—used to be a theater in Lame Deer. But we just stayed home many times—bead, or bake.

Here Vicky emphasizes ethics of hard work and self-sufficiency and conveys a sense of intergenerational continuity in how she learned crafts and other domestic skills from her mother and aunt. The importance of extended family is clear in how her cousin served as her close companion. She also describes the major recreation as exploring the local landscape, with only occasional public entertainment, such as dances. She does not mark tensions between Native and non-Native institutions and practices, describing how beadwork and "Indian"-style dances coexisted with activities at a local movie theater and the non-Native dance hall across the reservation line.

In a similarly structured account, Laura describes growing up in the vicinity of Lame Deer in an extended family household:

My dad always worked, always supported us. My mom kept house, sewed just about every day. She made quilts, and used to give them away to the elders at Christmas time. . . . We all went to Mennonite church. Thursday night sewing classes, prayer meeting Wednesday night, church Sunday night, vacation Bible school. When I was older I taught Sunday school and Bible summer school. My dad and two brothers had a singing group, a drum group. They would play for round dances, at powwows. They were really good, and popular. They didn't dance but just sang. I remember they would walk in the bitter cold to the dance hall—that's how much they liked to sing.

Here she emphasizes the propriety of men's roles as providers and women's roles as caregivers, as well as how giving away goods to elders enacted appropriate intergenerational respect. Like Vicky, Laura does not describe significant tension between Cheyenne and non-Native institutions and activities: Cheyenne drumming, singing, and giveaways coexist harmoniously with sewing quilts, observing Christian holidays, and participating in Bible school.

In these ways, older women's narratives convey that daily life was labor-intensive but cooperative, and how families enjoyed recreational activities together centered on home and community. As their narratives progressed, most then attributed the reproduction and maintenance of this harmonious and collaborative ethos to the cultivation of Cheyenne persons that are capable of participation in this distinctive ethical, behavioral, and affective world. Older women's accounts especially emphasize how kinship-based collaboration and intergenerational respect guided their development as children. Extended-family members all played roles in teaching and supervising children. Vivian summarizes the tenor of intergenerational relations in her childhood as follows: "Back then, there was always someone watching you." As Mary explains, children in this era fulfilled their proper role of listening (see also Straus 1977): "Our folks didn't really worry about us. We listened to our folks." Descriptions of various methods that parents, aunts, uncles, and grandparents used to cultivate such sensibilities often followed.

Cultivating Cheyenne Personhood: Teaching and Learning

Older women mention several common methods of discipline, including adults throwing a small amount of water on a temperamental child (to "cool them off"), and families cooperatively and temporarily excluding a misbehaving child from participation in family life. Many women also mention the disciplinarian roles of their maternal uncles, as Sara recounts with humor: "When I was real small, seems like my Uncle Joe was always there. If we did something wrong, my mom would say, 'I'll tell Uncle Joe.' It got so that I didn't much care for Uncle Joe!" [laughs].

Older women's accounts especially emphasize lessons in positive ethics that were aimed at promoting smooth social relationships. Some emphasize how they were taught by mothers, fathers, grandparents, and other caregivers not to invite conflict or trouble into their lives by lying, cheating, or stealing. Some also stress the importance of ethics of generosity, egalitarianism, and collective responsibility. As Vivian summarizes: "Never put yourself above your own people."

Many also recall how they were taught to speak carefully, and not to fuel existing social tensions by either engaging in or encouraging others' careless talk. As Sara says, "My dad taught us, 'Don't talk about other people, or get in on it if someone else is doing it. Don't repeat what someone else says about a person, since you don't know if it's true.'" Such teachings position the use of language and how one speaks as fundamental to personhood and sociality.

Older women's accounts also recurrently reference proper emotional expression as an essential feature of smooth social relations in their childhood lives. Laura praises her elderly grandfather's calm and pleasant demeanor in the face of the pain of a serious illness in his old age, for example, and remarks that though life was difficult and labor-intensive in her household, "no one complained." Others express special admiration for people who "never got mad" in response to interpersonal difficulties. Sara praises her grandfather's even temper and patient demeanor when her aunts would use up his money so that he could not buy groceries at the store, validating the maintenance of a calm and conflict-reducing demeanor even in the face of severe challenges.

Yet while emphasizing listening to and respecting the teaching of adults, older women's narratives of childhood do not valorize blind obedience to adult teachings or expectations. Instead, many depict childhood as a time to test or challenge rules set by adults, characterized (often with humor) as trying to "get away with something." Many describe fairly benign actions, like Vicky's story of how she and her cousin entered areas of the hills that her parents had warned her about: "We did find quite a few graves, too. We would always get scared and run away!" In such accounts, testing rules and limits is not necessarily transgressive in itself, but part of a cultural expectation that individuals cultivate a personalized understanding of why and how to abide by rules and limits.

In a similar vein, many older women comment that adult supervision sometimes placed unwelcome restrictions on their youthful activities. One recurrent example concerned older women's regulation of the sexual behavior of younger generations. As Sara describes:

My mother was strict with us girls—like we couldn't go out after dark. If we were at a dance at the dance hall in Lame Deer, we would go with my mother and my nephew. He was a tattletale! If we even stepped outside, we'd have to go home. My mother was strict—she told us if we ever stayed out all night with a boy, we would have to marry him. So we never had a lot of boyfriends. She'd stand right there so we couldn't hardly talk to them! As we got older, my mother wasn't so strict—we just had a curfew.

In one of many contrasts that older women drew between their early lives and the present conditions of reservation life, Sara went on to criticize younger women in the community for spending nights with their boyfriends, portraying the decline of these constraints as a loss, even though she experienced such restrictions as frustrating in her youth. Her comments therefore cast frustration as an element of youthful development, rather than a serious threat to cultural continuity across the generations. Yet some older women describe more profound discontent with adult interventions in their lives as youths. Vivian, an older Northern Cheyenne woman who spoke at several community workshops and gatherings in the mid-1990s, noted at a community recovery workshop in 1995: "There are a lot of 'don'ts' in traditional ways. My uncle used to come and talk to me, about Cheyenne culture, history, people. In those days, we had to sit there and listen when someone was talking to us. We couldn't talk back. I was always mad to see him! I would always think, 'Here he comes, to tell me more of those bad things.'" Vivian's point seems to be that at that age, she did not want to sit there and listen for long periods of time without being able to say anything—and especially, to hear about all of the limitations being placed upon her behavior. This story conveys an experience of deeper contradiction between being a Cheyenne person and participating in modern life. Yet in keeping with her current role as an elder, Vivian tells this story as a cautionary tale, ultimately emphasizing her later regrets about not listening and the consequences that she suffered. As such, her comments ultimately work to reinforce the need for adult supervision and teaching and the social authority of adults relative to youth.

Vivian's comment also invokes "tradition," a locally esteemed mode of asserting social authority. She describes receiving teachings and knowledge about traditional ways, even as she resisted. Yet a number of other older women's comments emphasize how adhering to tradition means respecting boundaries, and therefore actually not having access to specialized knowledge. Women's stories of experiences with ritual practices especially illustrate this point.

Respectful Relations: Other-than-Human Persons and Powers

In addition to social relationships within family and community, proper respect for Cheyenne spiritual beliefs and practices also figures prominently in older women's accounts of how personal and collective well-being was maintained in their childhood lives. Several women describe their awareness and acceptance of the importance of following various supernaturally sanctioned behavioral proscriptions. Vicky recounts:

> I remember my grandma doctoring an old lady. She was Indian doctor. You couldn't just go in front of her; had to go 'way around. A lady who had her menstrual period was not supposed to go around her or when someone was being doctored. And when you come out of a house where they been doctoring, you have to go in three, four, different places before you go back in, especially if it's dark outside. It's like purifying yourself of bad spirits, to do that.

Vicky describes recognizing and respecting the status of healers, and being cognizant of the danger inherent in the spiritual powers invoked by their activities.

Josephine produced a particularly rich description of how and why she learned from her grandmother to take supernatural proscriptions seriously:

> My grandma used to tell stories. People would bring chokecherries, Bull Durham, and all the village kids you know would sit around, and then she would tell us stories. She would tell us, "I don't want anybody interfering, I don't want anybody talking." You don't ever try to interrupt her, because she was like a medicine woman, she used to Indian doctor, deliver kids and all that. She said it was a gift that she had, that doctoring. She used to tell us to keep our friends away from that little house she lived in. 'Cause right in the back of it she had a big bundle, that medicine bag. And she said, "Don't stay around it, don't go around it, don't throw things at it." And boy, it was the way she raised us. To this day I still go by that—don't drag rope in the house, don't whistle in the house, don't play with knives, don't point knives at each other, don't stir with a knife when you're cooking. Don't play ball in the house. I still have that in me.

Here, Josephine portrays her grandmother as a wise and powerful person, in the eyes of the village and in her demonstrated healing power, lending credence to her teachings about the dangers inherent in disrespecting other-than-human powers. Her story also affirms the notion that a Cheyenne person is fundamentally constituted through listening to elders, and she claims her own entitlement to personhood by these standards by noting how she still has her grandmother's teachings "in me."

While older women's statements about direct personal experience with teachings about Cheyenne spiritual beliefs and practices vary, many do describe witnessing the strength of other-than-human powers in childhood. Rosemary recalls: "I used to always get pneumonia as a child. I was there in the new hospital for five months once. I remember one time I must have had a high fever, and I was talking to people who weren't there—delirious. My mother prayed for me. My mother was a praying woman. I got well." Others speak of times of hunger when families who had some food would cook and feed relatives and community members who did not, with several noting how medicine people would pray over the food and there seemed to always be just enough to go around.

Yet while conveying awareness and respect for local spiritual practitioners and practices, many older women's accounts convey a strong sense of distance from and/or incomplete knowledge of Cheyenne ritual practices. For example, Laura specifies that she did not learn the details of these practices. Instead, she learned that these ways were powerful and warranted respect by avoidance:

> My dad was sort of what you call a medicine man now. He danced five times in Sun Dance, but he was not a painter [a man who teaches and supervises dancers]. He knew his own design, but he never did it. Young guys would ask him, but he was really traditional and didn't participate. He had a lot of kids—didn't want any to get hurt. So he would just help set up the [Sun Dance] lodge. My mom told me to stay away—it was nothing to fool with. I respect it, so I stay away.

Laura notes how her father was "traditional" in exercising high levels of caution in ceremonial protocol, fearing consequences even if he used ritual powers that he had earned the right to exercise. She thereby constructs spiritual power as inherently dangerous and always possible to mismanage, and she invokes the advice and examples of both of her parents to justify her own avoidance of these practices.

In these ways, older women's narratives depict a Cheyenne world centered on family, community, and appropriate ritual relations with other-than-human powers. While this world is clearly embedded within non-Native society, their portraits highlight its distinctive local morality. Stories of specific encounters with non-Native institutions further emphasize this theme.

Churches and Schools: Threats Managed

In their narratives of childhood and adolescence, older women reference non-Natives largely through descriptions of their experiences at churches and schools. Both institutions pose clear potential threats to well-being in their accounts, but older women's narratives recurrently cast these threats as managed.

In Laura's account above, for example, the Mennonite church was integrated into the local world in the service of sustaining Cheyenne well-being. Yet Josephine describes Christian churches as a potential threat. In a characteristically rich description, she describes visiting two churches, guided by the pragmatic sensibilities of what each had to offer a child in search of entertainment:

> Sundays we would all go across there—right after [Catholic] mass, boy, we were speeding across to Mennonite church! [laughs] After services [the Mennonite minister's wife] would let us play the piano, and she would have guitars, and every once in a while she would have a bonfire in the evening [with] wieners and marshmallows. Pretty soon this one priest came along, and I guess he heard what was going on! [laughs] I don't know who told him. . . . And finally this priest kind of said, "If you're gonna come to Catholic church, you stick with the Catholic church, you're Catholic. You cannot run across to the Mennonite church." He said, "Catholic church is the one true church." And you know, that's confusing. He confused me. And I told my grandma, I said, "Grandma," I said, "There's two Gods, Catholics have one, and Mennonites have one." And I said, "Which one, which one is true?" She said, "The true God is the one we know and understand, so we pray to one God." She said, "I pray. I'm a Cheyenne. We have peyote meetings. We go in there, sit up all night, pray and sing." And she said, "You go to two churches, you pray. You pray to the same God.

To me it's good that you go to church twice. Because you got to start believing [in God]. Don't let them confuse you."

Here, Josephine emphasizes how her grandmother role-modeled an effective synthesis, placing the highest value on the broad goals of learning the practice of prayer and cultivating a sense of faith. She clearly communicated that quibbling about how simply introduces needless confusion, helping Josephine to avoid this threat to her well-being.

Numerous references to school also appear in older women's accounts, with similar rhetorical themes of how threats to Cheyenne well-being were managed. As Mary recalls, for example:

I started school when I was eight or nine years old. We went to boarding school. I think my family couldn't support us. I really wanted to be with my folks—I used to get lonesome for them. I liked living at home, out in the country. We stayed at school on weekdays and sometimes weekends, if our folks were in Sheridan. I liked being in the dorms. I heard that older generations were beaten for talking Cheyenne at Mission and at Lame Deer school, but I don't remember any of that. I remember that I didn't like to eat Jell-O, and the matron turned hot water on and pushed us in the shower, to punish us. I told on her once, and my brother wanted to fight her. So, she stopped. That was the only bad experience I had there.

Beating and pushing contrast sharply with the methods of discipline that women recalled from earlier childhood, underscoring both their foreignness and harmfulness. Yet, while acknowledging these techniques of forced assimilation, Mary denies suffering harm from them. Laura offers a similar account:

Mother had been to school and knew how to speak, read, and write English; but my dad did not know, or my grandparents. I didn't know English until third grade. I remember before that, Teacher got mad at me, shook me. I didn't understand. Turned out she was accusing me of stealing. I didn't even know anything about it. Mother went and talked for me—she really got after that teacher! That was the end of that—that teacher never did bother me again. And I started school at Mission in 1952. . . . Mission used to have a bakery, with homemade bread, milk, and butter. I used to work there. We would eat bread and butter, dip it into the milk. The little ones would knock on the window or door if they were hungry, and we would give them bread through there. If we got caught, we were in trouble! The nuns were mean.

Like Mary, Laura references feelings of loneliness, the foreignness of school, and the sometimes intimidating tactics employed by authority figures there. Yet both women's narratives ultimately emphasize their management and resolution of these conflicts, with Mary appealing to her brother's, and Laura to her mother's, protective role.

In these ways, older women discursively construct a kinship-centered moral universe populated by grandmothers, mothers, brothers, and others in their early childhood lives that mitigated potentially harmful interactions with non-Natives. As topics turned to early memories of alcohol, however, this theme of threats managed began to be replaced by imagery of erosion and decline.

Accounts of Drinking: Rhetorics of Moral Erosion

As one might expect, older women interested in sobriety made numerous general comments about the changes wrought by the marked rise of drinking circa midcentury on the reservation. Examples include: "We enjoyed just being together. There was no drugs or alcohol" (Rosemary); "We had fun without drinking or drugs. Sun Dances, hand games, Indian dances" (Mary); "Seems like they never mentioned any drinking during that time—no smoking marijuana or anything like that. They talked about powwows and Sun Dance" (Laura). These comments contrast a world of fuller engagement with Cheyenne cultural heritage, and a higher moral value, with the world of today, in which many social relationships and recreational practices in the community are centered on substances.

Yet placing these comments in the context of older women's broader life history narratives suggests that their accounts do not make quite clear the role of alcohol as a causal factor in this moral decline. Upon close reading, alcohol rhetorically figures as a symptom of a broader process: initially manageable within a coherent moral world, but then unmanageable, transgressive of that world's ethics and values as the latter were already beginning to deteriorate.

Early Memories of Alcohol: Management

As in their discussions of churches and schools above, some older women's accounts of their earliest memories acknowledge the rise of alcohol but rhetorically contain its negative consequences. Esther emphasizes how her uncle drank but continued to maintain locally esteemed standards of comportment and skill: "My uncle . . . got accustomed to drinking in Europe in World War I. He kept using when he got back. I saw that growing up—but I never saw him stagger, use profanity, or get really drunk. He always had a very reserved, civil manner with people. And he was a good singer—he was invited to powwows. He never lost his language." Here she stresses that alcohol played a minor role in her uncle's life. Similarly, Vicky describes how her dad drank but continued to fulfill his role as provider for the family: "When I was a teenager the only one I seen drinking in my home was my dad. But he was working all the time, too. He just drank sometimes, like at dances or on weekends. He held down a job."

These types of comments assert that Cheyenne personhood was fundamentally maintained in face of the threat to well-being posed by rising alcohol use. Many older women reiterate these themes as they discuss their own entry into alcohol use. A number recount drinking with largely female groups of friends, with no serious or unpleasant consequences beyond feeling sick or hung over the next day. In Laura's words: "A friend of mine in high school would get wine for us. At first it was OK, and then I started having really bad hangovers. So then I started with beer. There were just girls our age at these parties—we would go swimming, drink beer. We had fun." Such stories give no indication that drinking resulted in transgressions of the patterns of thought, feeling, or behavior inculcated in earlier childhood.

Yet many older women also describe witnessing a profound transition in the impact of alcohol, locating a point in time within their early lives at which drinking became a markedly destructive force. Key examples in these stories center on the disruption of social relationships within household and community.

Beyond Management: Alcohol's Transgressive Power

Vicky recounts how the prevalence of alcohol use began to affect community activities in her adolescence:

They would have Indian dances. My folks were pretty involved in that, and even us kids were on the planning committee. The dance would be going on, real good, and then drunks would start coming over—younger ones. They would try to pick a fight, and pretty soon break up the activity. The cops would come over, and that was the end of the dance. Quite a few would come in drunk to dances in Lame Deer. They would interfere with the singing. And they used to put a horse by the door, so nobody could go out. It's like a bet—you can't open the door unless somebody bets a horse against it. So, everyone has to stay and dance all night. . . . People would be mad. Like us, we came a long way, and the little kids would be tired. We used to be mad. But even the cops couldn't do anything about it.

This story emphasizes how drinking led to spurious abuses of local practices. Here, Vicky also conveys that this new threat to well-being was unprecedented, and not amenable to management.

A number of women also describe witnessing a transition within their families, as their parents and/or siblings began to take up drinking. Mary says: "We were one of the families that went out to pick sugar beets. All the families would buy beer and drink. I had never seen my folks drunk, so I would cry. I didn't want them to drink. They used to tell us [earlier when I was] growing up, 'Drinking families are no good, not worth it, nobody cares for them.' Like they were always looked down on. I think I really remembered that." Mary describes directly witnessing a profound change in the rising acceptance of drinking in new segments of the community. Similarly, Laura's account of her later childhood includes a marked shift in tone, describing how alcohol fueled transgressions of the collaborative and protective relationships within her natal family:

My dad had a friend who liked to drink. On weekends they would go drink, and my dad would be the chauffeur. He would come home late and drunk. . . . My dad would go to sleep and be hung over all day Sunday, but then be back at work Monday. When I was away in school, then he started taking my mother with him more. I remember this from summertimes. We used to go with them, maybe go to Sheridan. They would be all right until they saw some friends, and then would want to go drink. So after a while we didn't want to go [with them], and we'd stay home with our grandparents. We missed them. Then my dad started getting mad, raising hell with my mom.

Or he'd wake up the kids, make them sit up in the middle of the night to talk to them. Didn't make any sense, what he was saying. Then he'd say, "Go back to sleep!" He was a mean guy; we all listened to him.

Laura's description of "we missed them" and of her father being "mean" mark a dramatic departure from the moral configuration of her earlier world. Alcohol figures as a central and regrettable element in this change.

The notion that moral erosion accompanied the rise of drinking emerges most vividly in older women's accounts of alcohol-related violence. Vicky describes observing a rise in alcohol-related violence among neighboring families in the Birney area: "There were some men who would drink and run out their family. They would run to neighbors to stay for the night. We used to have quite a few stay with us. The men never came to look for them—just stayed away. Usually [the family] would go back home next day." Other women describe witnessing violence within their own households. Faith recounts a particularly dramatic instance from growing up in Busby:

My older brother and his friends used to come home drunk, wake us up—fighting. We'd run out with no shoes on, scared that he would hit us. Sleep at a neighbor's. I didn't like it. My mom said, "You should go drink somewhere else." Then one time he got mad, said he would beat up Old Man. Old Man ran out. So he beat up my mom instead. That really hurt me. I never forgot that; it still bothers me. He came back, he was quiet. I don't know how he felt, but she had a black eye and swollen face. I didn't see him apologize or anything.

The intergenerational character of this assault is especially salient, given the value placed upon respectful relations between parents and children that older women's accounts emphasize. Faith's emotional response to this disturbing attack is strong ("it still bothers me . . ."), and she portrays her inability to discern her brother's emotional or social reaction as part of the reason why. From her perspective, it seems, her brother's violence has positioned him outside the parameters of intelligible Cheyenne personhood.

In these excerpts, older women primarily offer examples of male alcohol-related violence. Sara notes that some women in her childhood town of Busby did drink, however, and that they became violent: "This one

woman, a real mean woman, would get drunk and go out and terror-
ize people. There were two families that drank, too—they both had a lot
of kids, and the women would really fight. Everyone would watch!" Yet
the overwhelming majority of older women's stories about violence portray men as its perpetrators and emphasize how women and children
suffered the consequences. Gender therefore figures in their stories as a
prominent site of moral disruption due to alcohol use.

Gender, Alcohol, and Moral Erosion

Older women generally offer fairly nonspecific descriptions of violence,
such as hitting, like Faith's story above. Only a few mention alcohol-
related sexual violence. These stories are never personal, and with few
exceptions women did not raise them independently, but in response
to a question from me. The most explicit story was volunteered by
Josephine:

> My friend used to drink. She didn't come home that one time. Here
> they found her out in the hills, no clothes on. She got in with a group
> of guys, her and another girl. That other girl came home by herself,
> and that's when they found my friend next day. She was all naked. She
> had been beaten up too. Her hair was sticky, stiff; they poured liquor
> on her hair. My grandma told her, and told us, not to go around those
> guys. They would come around, and she would tell us we better just
> go home—stay away from them.

Note how here again too, Josephine portrays her grandmother as a wise
and authoritative figure, in informing girls about the serious threat that
these men posed.

Josephine is one of the more unusual figures in this study, since she
was born in the 1930s and so fits in the "older generation" category but
in the 1970s helped to found the first Alcoholics Anonymous group specifically for Northern Cheyenne women. Her more open discussion of
problems such as sexual abuse may reflect her greater familiarity with
Twelve Step conventions of openly discussing such experiences to emotionally come to terms with them.

Most other stories of alcohol-related sexual violence in older women's
narratives are less explicit. Many women remark that such instances were
infrequent. As Anne says, she initially thought that child molestation

was something that happened only in the non-Native world: "I never heard about sexual abuse and child molesting on the reservation, when I was small. Then when I got big, I would read or hear about it out there—I thought it was just white people. [On the reservation] there was just one guy, they told us to watch out for—he had raped somebody. Everyone was so scared of him." Other women note a prevailing understanding among adults in their early lives that sexual abuse was related to drinking and rose in correlation with it. Vicky comments: "It had something to do with alcohol. My parents and grandfolks told me 'If they're drinking, they don't know what they're doing.'" Mary echoed this theme, saying, "My grandmother and my mother would tell us . . . don't be around your brothers if they're drinking—they don't know what they're doing. Stay away from anybody that's drinking.'" Local understandings of drunkenness as a "time out" from normal social expectations seem evident here.

Alcohol's disruption of women's abilities to manage the sexual behavior of men is especially transgressive in light of the emphasis so much ethnographic material places upon Cheyenne women's responsibilities for sexual regulation; the transgressive effects of alcohol on gender roles and relations include eroding women's abilities to manage the sexual behavior of men. Here too, older women seem to portray alcohol as profoundly altering personhood: men are fundamentally not themselves while drinking, and "don't know what they're doing." While "crazy" behavior that violates core moral values of Cheyenne behavior is seen as part of the human condition in prominent Cheyenne ethnopsychological theories, these women's narratives emphasize the consequences that such behavior has for others. Such talk reflects the importance of women's social roles in negatively sanctioning such behavior. But significantly too these excerpts convey how a time arrived at which such sanctioning was no longer effective. Their comments indicate that not much could be done about these transgressions, beyond minimizing their damage through awareness and avoidance.

Summary: Older Women's Rhetoric

When asked about their early memories and about the impact of alcohol on their childhood and adolescent lives, older women tell strikingly detailed stories about the nature of Cheyenne personhood and its contribution to a coherent and constructive moral world in their early lives. They clearly position themselves as witnesses to major changes in reservation life and emphasize the high moral worth of a past now gone. The fact that the Cheyenne world was embedded within the non-Native world, with the associated social inequalities and imposed values, is acknowledged but rhetorically managed and contained in their accounts. Their narratives center heavily on description of changes rather than explicit explanation, recurrently emphasizing how their early lives were "not like now." Prominent local rhetorical conventions that construct a past era as a moral center that no longer does or can fully exist seem evident here.

By not offering an explicit explanation of why these transformations occurred, while identifying alcohol as a central factor, one could conclude that older women see alcohol as the primary cause of the decline of Cheyenne personhood. But continuing analysis of their narratives suggests a more complex reading, in which alcohol figures more as a symptom of a broader process. Before considering these issues, however, a contrast with younger women's discussions of their childhoods illuminates key differences in the historical experiences of Northern Cheyenne women's early lives, and in the rhetorical tools that women use to represent their personal histories.

Younger Women: Drinking as Collective History

Rather than describing a decline from a period of coherence in their early lives, most younger women's narratives centrally emphasize disruptive and painful experiences. Alcohol figures prominently as a direct cause of these troubling problems. All younger women also use at least some terms and concepts from Twelve Step approaches to recovery, including frequent references to "alcoholism," "dysfunction," "abuse," "abandonment" and "inner child."

Even so, prominent local rhetorical conventions also seem salient for younger women, who make numerous statements that morally privilege the past in general and/or specific Cheyenne cultural values and practices. Yet while these statements hold some similarity to older women's, upon closer examination younger women's ideas about "tradition" and the sources of authority that they reference are often quite different.

In what is perhaps a testament to the increasing diversity of social identities and/or rhetorical tools used by Northern Cheyenne community members after 1950, younger women's accounts of their early childhood lives include more variation than older women's. Some are entirely dominated by descriptions of alcohol-related abuse and neglect, with several women producing no other salient memories in an interview even when prompted. Most typical, however, are prevailing themes of alcohol-related disruption and pain, interwoven with occasional and brief but clearly significant stories about learning valued knowledge and skills.

Stories of Childhood: Pride, Confusion, and Pain

Brief stories of positive experiences in early childhood often highlight what the speaker finds to be particularly valuable about her Cheyenne cultural heritage. For example, a number of younger women who speak Cheyenne emphasize how much they value knowing it. Jenny explains:

> One of the really important things to me that I learned from my parents and my grandmother and my grandfather was our language, the Cheyenne language. It was instilled in us as children, and we just grew up with it, and there was even a time where we only knew each other by our Indian names. As we got into grade school, then we had to learn our English names. I'm really proud to be able to speak it and understand it. I don't really understand the real technical language, but I know the basic language and am able to pray in my language.

Jenny notes her pride in knowing Cheyenne, especially given its decline within her own and subsequent generations of community members. Her statements of pride in knowing it and about being "able to pray in my language" also indicate how both language and ritual practices serve as key signifiers of Cheyenne identity in contemporary reservation social life, as ethnographers document in other reservation communities (see also Gone 2006; O'Nell 1996).

In a parallel fashion to older women, younger women also tell stories of witnessing the power of local ritual healing practices as children. Heather described being diagnosed with a spinal problem that doctors felt required surgery, but which resolved and required no medical intervention after her grandparents held a peyote meeting for her. Such stories convey both the vitality and the impact of local cultural resources in younger women's childhood lives.

Other younger women describe other positive memories of learning valued skills. Grandparents figure as key teachers in these stories, with most parents temporarily or permanently absent due to active drinking or alcohol-related deaths. As Louise, Theresa, and Jeanne variously describe:

> I stayed with my grandmother more than with my parents. The things I remember about my parents are just bars, drinking. But with my grandma, we used to come in here [by the river] to cut twigs and spread our blanket out on the ground. You know, I was just small. We'd carry [wood] on our backs. We would pick chokecherries and wild turnips, and then mushrooms after it rained. Sometimes catch and cook turtle. (Louise)

> [When my parents went on a drinking binge, then they] would leave us with my grandparents. That's way out in the middle of nowhere, but, you know, thinking back on it, I remember it being real peaceful, and we could do whatever we wanted; we could spend time in the hills or go get the horses, and we'd ride the horses. And then, like, whenever the berries would get ripe, we'd pick berries and plums, you know. Or my grandpa would hunt and get deer and we'd help fix that. I really cherish those thoughts sometimes. I just sit and think about it, it is so clean, peaceful, green, and, you know, to me that was the life. (Theresa)

> I'm really thankful that [my grandparents] raised me. I always think that if they hadn't raised me, I would have never spoke Cheyenne. We used to go to powwows, we used to dance, and, like, we were into horses, you know, like a ranch, we did that, and then my grandfather was one where they pierce, out in the hills? And peyote meetings, he did that too. So we always kind of did everything, you know? And I'm really thankful for that. Because I know a little of something. (Jeanne)

In these ways, like older women, younger women clearly identify elements that they associate with Cheyenne cultural heritage and imbue them with positive moral value. Yet differences are also evident. Jeanne sets forth a well-rounded person as an ideal by emphasizing the importance of being acquainted with the variety of distinct local lifeways, including powwow dancing, ranching and rodeo, Cheyenne ritual practices (fasting and piercing), and peyote meetings. Such flexibility is not as explicitly discussed by older women, whose narratives focus

instead on a more circumscribed set of teachings, ethics, and comportment. Different ways of defining and evaluating Cheyenne personhood
are apparent here.

While some younger women describe spending substantive time
with elders such as grandparents, these accounts also contrast with older
women's. Some younger women strikingly position their childhood
selves as spectators rather than participants in the world of their elders.
For instance, Becky's recollections of her grandmother read as discrete
scenes and details:

> And my grandmother—she was a traditional Indian woman, med-
> icine woman. I remember when I was really little, must have been
> seven and eight, I was in a sweat with them, the first sweat I remem-
> ber being in. Them old ladies used to come over there and make dry
> meat and sing Indian songs. And I just remember being out there, it
> was really something. They used to wear those old Indian bandan-
> nas? Around their heads like this? [gestures] And they used to cut
> dry meat and sing Indian songs. They had these cute little laughs. You
> know, those old Indian people—I can still see my grandma out there,
> laughing like those old Indian people; they were just cute. I spent a lot
> of time down there when my mom and dad used to drink.

Although her affection and admiration for her grandmother emerge
clearly here, so too does a sense that Becky herself was a rather disconnected observer of these scenes. Statements concerning what "those old
Indian people" wore, what they did, and how they sounded contrast with
the narratives of older women like Josephine, who clearly portrayed her
grandmother as an active caregiver in Josephine's daily life as a child.
Language barriers account at least in part for this difference, since Becky
is among the many younger-generation women who did not grow up
learning to speak Cheyenne.

Indeed, throughout our interactions, Becky has frequently referenced
her struggles to learn more about her heritage, not speaking Cheyenne
and identified as a "half-breed." She also describes recurrent frustrations
with how people who were raised to speak Cheyenne and/or are considered "full-bloods" fail to appreciate what she did learn while growing up or later through her own efforts. Other younger women's narratives of childhood similarly focus on experiences of social exclusion and

other painful experiences, and frequently connect these to alcohol-rlated family dynamics and experiences of violence.

Instability, Placelessness, and Confusion

Rather than the stable kinship-centered world depicted in older women's accounts, younger women describe experiences of frequent moves, changing caregivers, and domestic violence. Experiences of community exclusion, and the disruptions of illness and imprisonment of caregivers or other family members, also appear far more frequently in their accounts. While younger women do not universally attribute all of these problems to alcohol, they frequently connect them to drinking. For example, Ellen positions alcohol as a central cause of violence and other disruptions in her early experiences: "I was aware of alcohol at an early age. There was violence. My mother was abused in her marriage by my father, and it was usually when he was intoxicated. The other incidents concerning [other relatives] . . . were just crazy things that would happen that made our life kind of crazy. You know, they'd come home, be sick all through the day, or they'd be in jail."

Younger women's narratives also include far more emphasis on the emotional dimensions of their experiences. In keeping with Twelve Step conventions, prominent among these are feelings of fear, anger, shame, and resulting difficulties that powerfully disrupted their development from childhood to adulthood. For instance, Jenny offers the following account of how alcohol contributed to family disruption in her childhood after her father died from drinking and his family blamed her mother for his death and threatened her life to keep her away from the children: "It was really ugly, and we were just little kids, and that was the hardest thing for me . . . so we suffered some more abandonment issues, and we kind of got thrown around between aunties and uncles and different people, relatives. But the people that were taking care of us were all alcoholic families . . . [until] finally my grandfather got custody over us." In this account of intense conflict and the pain that it caused her as a child, Jenny clearly draws upon ACOA terms and concepts like "abandonment issues" and "alcoholic families."

In addition to deaths and conflicts, unclaimed paternity figures as a key disruption to family and kinship in younger women's accounts. While not unknown among older women, this problem is far more frequently referenced and discussed by younger women and is often linked with alcohol use. In drinking situations on the reservation, children are sometimes conceived in a one-time encounter between people who do not otherwise have a relationship, for example. Sometimes an encounter is considered embarrassing and/or is not talked about, since it involves an unknown or unremembered partner or people who are related by the terms of the Cheyenne kinship system, since one or both of the parents are (or later became) married to other people, or since it involved sexual violence.

Karen's parents met while drinking, and her father refused to claim paternity. Her mother then remarried a man who drank heavily. Karen describes how she confronted the fact of her lack of place in reservation social structure in trying to manage this situation.

> My stepdad really used. And there was times when I would have to run down to my stepdad's grandmother's and hide, and my step-grandmother didn't like me. She was saying, "You got your own grandma. I'm not your grandma." But that was after my grandma had died, and I had no place to go. So I had no choice but to stay there and just take it. And I was always called a bastard, ever since I can remember. "You're a bastard. . . . I know your dad and your dad don't care for you."

Stories of conflicts based on degree of Cheyenne "blood," even though they were usually not as explicitly related to alcohol, were also frequent in younger women's narratives and rhetorically parallel stories of unclaimed paternity, by including similarly intense accounts of feelings of exclusion.

All younger women describe other painful family dynamics related to alcohol, and how these disrupted their personal development. Their accounts corroborate the changes in family and community life that older women described from the 1950s onward, yet reflect a distinct set of rhetorical tools for representing these experiences by focusing explicitly and at length on their psychological dimensions.

Narrative Focus: The Psychological Impact of Alcohol

Younger women offer detailed accounts of painful emotional experiences that stemmed from their parents' drinking. These include feelings of being unwanted or abandoned, having their basic needs and safety neglected, and being prematurely forced to take on adult responsibilities.

Andrea describes: "My parents drank. I don't know how old I was when they quit, but I always got left behind. [They would] find different babysitters and leave me with them or lock me up in the house and just go party. [I felt like my mother] didn't want me." As quoted in chapter 1, Becky describes waiting for her parents outside bars for hours in a hot car. At another point in her narrative of childhood, she elaborates:

> All the time that I was in boarding school, all the time I was there—I was there 13 years—I cannot remember my mom and dad coming to visit me. That's how it was. And all my siblings were there, but I never ever remember them coming to visit me. We just felt really abandoned and dumped. They drank most of the time; when I was little they were binge drinkers. There was a lot of fear when I was younger, you know, when the weekend was coming I used to fear coming home on that bus, because I knew they wouldn't be home. I really used to cry, and pray, that maybe—I used to think if there was a God in heaven, let them be home, and there was a point in my life when I hated God because they weren't home. There wasn't no God in my life. Gee—that must have been third, fourth grade?

Theresa offers a highly similar account of the emotional pain of neglect, also noting its pragmatic problems, such as when her father would get paid and spend the money on alcohol for the parents rather than on food or other necessities for the children. As a result, unwanted caregiving tasks fell to her: "I'm the oldest daughter in the family, and it was kind of up to me to take care of the little ones. I was the mom, I was taking care of the little ones. I didn't want to be a mom that young."

Both Becky and Theresa articulate intense desires for their parents' presence and care. Their efforts to pray and hope that things would be better, accompanying disappointment when they were not, and feeling of being forced to grow up too quickly take center stage. These themes are also prominent in Twelve Step constructions of ACOA experiences and problems of codependency, and at other points both Becky and Theresa demonstrate their familiarity with these constructs by using the term "inner child" to describe how these experiences disrupted their development.

Many younger women also tell stories of childhood that go beyond neglect to describe more extreme forms of violence. When I asked, Laurie replied that she simply could not recall any memories of her childhood beyond drinking, violence, and various forms of abuse by her family members. She describes feeling so overloaded with negative emotion and stress as a child that she became numb as a way of coping. Becky also depicts witnessing her parents come home drunk, fighting and threatening to kill each other, as an all-encompassing experience that required intense psychological energy: "so whenever they would drink, we would have to hide everything, you know, hide all the guns and all the knives and, you know, anything sharp. And that violence is so powerful that it's just paralyzing. You know, you just had to prepare yourself for when they were drinking." "Paralyzing" conveys the intensity of emotion involved, and how the realities and constant threat of such experiences diverted energy from other childhood needs.

Many of the most evocative uses of language and visible displays of emotion during the interviews accompanied younger women's descriptions of sexual abuse during childhood and adolescence. Recall that in their accounts, older women recognize sexual violence and relate it to alcohol but do not describe it as widespread or in terms of personal experiences. Younger women are far more likely to talk explicitly about such experiences, in part reflecting their familiarity and involvement with the disclosure practices of Twelve Step therapies.

Numerous studies document the troubling prevalence of sexual violence against Native North American women, and the profound gaps in legal responses and limited community resources for preventing such violence or assisting survivors (e.g., Smith 2005). While younger women often explicitly link experiences of sexual assault in adolescence with alcohol (see below), those who describe experiences of sexual abuse in earlier childhood often did not specify whether alcohol was involved. Nonetheless, younger women clearly weave stories of childhood sexual abuse into their larger narratives of alcohol's impact on their lives, by describing how the emotional pain of these experiences often contributed to their own later drinking patterns.

Stories of sexual abuse in childhood range from one event with one perpetrator, to multiple events with one perpetrator, to multiple events with a number of different perpetrators. Women describe the majority of perpetrators as male, although some make references to females as well. Many were relatives but some were not, including neighbors and friends of the family. Most were Native, but some of the latter were non-Native. Most perpetrators were adults, but some were other chil-

dren, often slightly older children who had often, as some women later
learned, been victims of sexual abuse themselves.

Women frequently describe responding to these experiences with
intense feelings of anger. Some direct anger at particular individuals—
oftentimes the perpetrator, although sometimes their responses to him
or her are mixed with other feelings (especially if that person was a relative). People who should have known or been available to help also figure as targets for these feelings (see also Herman 1992). Karen expresses
how she felt especially angry toward her mother: "To this day I've never
told my mother [that I was sexually abused by one of her boyfriends].
I believe in my heart that my mother had to know. A mother can feel a
child's pain, because I know I can feel my [children's] pain. I hated my
mother for not protecting me." Others describe directing more generalized anger toward the world. Andrea says: "I took a lot of anger out
on my mom, a lot of anger out on a lot of people that didn't even know
what was going on. I didn't know what to do with all that anger. I would
go to my room and just tear it apart. Take it out on my little sisters. Take
it out on other people." Alice, who describes being sexually abused for
most of her childhood and adolescence by a slightly older male relative,
describes the intense stress of living one's daily life in the presence of a
predator. She notes how she directed her feelings of anger toward God,
saying, "I refused to believe in a God that would let that happen."

Women portray the consequences of such experiences as profound,
and themselves as entering adolescence with serious disruptions in their
relationships with family, peers, and spiritual powers. They portray these
problems as intensifying as they went on in later childhood and early
adolescence to start drinking themselves.

Normative Drinking and Disrupted Development

Younger women's stories of their own involvements with alcohol range
widely, linking the genesis of their own drinking to the influence of
peers, the normative quality of drinking in reservation social life, and/or
the emotional pain experienced in childhood. While many of these link-
ages are also drawn in Twelve Step approaches, these do not generally
deal with the special challenges posed by the community-wide prevalence of drinking.

All younger women describe drinking on the reservation as prevalent, if not within their families, then definitely within their peer groups

in adolescence. Most describe how they started drinking in childhood, often with either implicit approval or open assistance from adult relatives. Jackie recounted how drinking was a family affair, centered on female kin and off-reservation bars: "I used to drink with my aunt. We'd go after chicken feed in Hardin and park in front of the bar, hit skid row, and just drink here and there. It was fun—I was with my favorite aunt, and with my cousin and about four other girls." Louise and Theresa describe learning to drink in the context of their households, following the example of adults:

> It was there, so we just drank it too. One time I found this cute little bottle. I didn't know what it was, but it must have been wine. And we were drinking it—I and my little sister, and we was playing on like these old wagons, big wagons that horses pulled. I don't know how old I was, but I think that's when I first felt different, you know? Like I started getting dizzy. (Louise)

> I can't remember when I started drinking. I was very young. The way it started is when my parents were drinking, we would steal their wine or their beer. And then it got to a point where they would buy, you know, their booze, they would buy beer for us. It was for us older kids. And maybe that was their way of kind of saying that it was all right to drink. . . . [My aunt and uncle] would let us use the car to run around in. We'd be out in the hills, partying, you know; that was a natural, normal thing to do. (Theresa)

These stories of early exposure to and active facilitation of drinking by caregivers depart markedly from those of older women, who referenced adult bootleggers in their stories of youthful drinking but emphasized how they consumed alcohol only occasionally and with groups of peers. While younger women also describe the influence of peers in their initiation to alcohol and other substance use, they portray the frequency of use as much higher, and the pressure to participate as much greater. Their stories especially feature siblings, cousins, and friends. Jeanne describes: "I was about 7th grade. There used to be a bunch of us girls that ran around together. We all tried everything!" [laughs] From sniffing fingernail polish and spray paint, they went on to try alcohol: "We drank out in the hills; it was just like drinking beer; somebody eventually would buy it for us. Somebody older, an older guy or somebody, and we'd go someplace. We kept on doing it, it was just something to do. There was always about six of us. . . . We'd go to Hardin or KS [Kirby Saloon, across the reservation line south of Busby]. We would all drink, and we went through it as like a phase or something." Similarly, Lynn recalls: "I think I was about ten. Most of my friends were older than me, and I saw them sipping on Coke and whiskey, or getting into their folks' beer and sneak it off somewhere. And I'd taste it. I didn't like that taste of it, but it was just so normal to do 'cause that's what everybody was doing, you know?" These excerpts clearly convey that substance use, centered on alcohol but by the 1960s including other drugs too, was a major form of recreation on the reservation by the time of younger women's childhood and young adult lives.

Many younger women relate their drinking with peers to their general desire for a social life in adolescence. Kim recalls, "In high school I went along because everyone was there—it was the thing to do! Even if you weren't drinking, going to parties was the thing to do. Your only other choice was to sit at home by yourself." Many note how alcohol use was often associated with meeting members of the opposite sex, as Theresa describes: "Sometimes we would run away from school, and we would drink. Sometimes we would crawl out the window to go meet some boys or, you know, have them get booze for us—that sort of thing. Well, we'd get caught sometimes, and we'd get in trouble, but most of the time we didn't get caught!"

Yet within this normative prevalence, younger women also describe variability in their own patterns of alcohol use. At one end of the spectrum, Becky describes drinking relatively little: "That was kind of my lifestyle of drinking. I would never really get drunk. I only remember getting drunk twice in my life. I went on parties, and of course I used to be the designated driver. I did my share of drinking. But I didn't enjoy it. I would have flashbacks of things that went on [in my parents' home], and I didn't like it." Younger women who discuss this style and who are familiar with Twelve Step concepts tend to describe themselves as codependent rather than alcoholic. At the other end, women like Laurie describe a much heavier style of active drinking: "I was a heavy user by sixteen or seventeen. It started out partying once a month, and then it quickly went to twice a month, and it was twice a month for three months, and then it just went to every week—where I was looking for a party every week."

Most younger women offer detailed psychological portraits of how and why they drank, in keeping with the Twelve Step conceptualization of "cycles," in which emotions of anger and grief lead to drinking, which produces consequences that create more anger and grief and lead to more drinking.

Psychological Motives for Drinking

Some women specifically relate their participation in peer drinking groups to neglect by their caretakers, later bolstered by resentment.

> My folks had divorced, so I was pretty much on my own 'cause I was living with grandma, and she was working, she was busy. Everybody was busy, so I just hung out with friends all the time. And then it got to every weekend that's what we did, even during the school year, every weekend that's what we did. We went out and we partied. From nine years old I was literally on my own, no one there, and by the time [my family] wanted to take control of me, I couldn't be controlled. By then I was bigger, and I'd challenge [them]—"Go ahead. Hit me." (Lynn)

Some women's accounts go further, to present themselves as reaching adulthood profoundly traumatized by childhood, and as motivated by the continuing salience of these feelings to drink heavily. Andrea describes an all-consuming response to years of sexual abuse: "I wanted to forget about it. I just basically wanted to crawl into a dark hole and drink myself to death."

Yet in a particularly vicious cycle, drinking also places young women at risk for sexual assault. Laurie describes how as a young teenager she was raped by an uncle, who got her drunk before assaulting her. Many other women identify drinking parties with their adolescent peers as key sites of risk, especially if a woman passed out from drinking. Sexual assault in these situations has been documented on the reservation and discussed with concern by a variety of community members since at least the 1970s (e.g., Straus 1976:212). Some younger women express a generalized awareness of this danger, with Carol commenting: "I was so scared to get drunk. We heard terrible stories about women getting drunk, and being sexually abused. I was always scared of that." Others, like Julie, tell personal stories of these experiences.

After I graduated high school, I was always at a party out of town. I met this one guy, and we were going together, and I don't even remember anything, but the next morning when I woke up, I noticed that I must have had sex that night, but I don't remember that part. But I got pregnant from that. I never even told [the father] that I got pregnant. I didn't really know him that much. And I just didn't want him to know, because I hated him for what he had done.

Marla describes how as a teenager she was gang-raped by a group of boys after she passed out at a drinking party—an experience whose acute trauma was intensified through boasting among the boys involved and gossip by other community members. Women's emotional responses to these experiences during our conversations were visible and understandably intense.

Experiences of alcohol-related sexual assault in young adulthood were isolated incidents for some women but served to compound the trauma of childhood sexual abuse for others. Younger women therefore portray sexuality and associated gender relations as an especially potent site for the disruptive effects of alcohol in their childhood and adolescence. While this theme broadly echoes older women's narratives, younger women's detailed descriptions of sexual trauma lend far more intensity to these concerns in their accounts.

Non-Native World: Ambivalence

Given how younger women portray numerous serious threats to well-being within their households, families, and communities in their early lives, their narratives neither follow older women's tendencies to morally compartmentalize the Cheyenne world against the non-Native world surrounding it nor to portray a relatively smooth integration of selected institutions such as schools and Christian churches into this Cheyenne world. Instead of such clarity, non-Native individuals and institutions figure in a highly ambivalent mixture of strongly negative and strongly positive capacities in younger women's narratives.

For example, younger women explicitly discuss how being embedded within non-Native society and subjected to special policies such as tribal enrollment disrupted their well-being as children. Some report experiences of harsh teasing and exclusion for being enrolled members of other tribes, even though they were raised on the reservation by their Cheyenne relatives. Several recall how they were raised with one side of their family multiethnic, and the other side Cheyenne. Each side severely criticized the other, producing considerable feelings of confusion, as Lynn describes: "The one side said that if I took up the beliefs of the other side, then I would go to hell instead of heaven. That really scared me. And the other side said, 'White people took our land, they cheated and lied to us, and they are always telling us that our ways are bad. Don't listen to them.' I was always confused by that. I loved them both, but they hated each other. As a little girl, I didn't know what to do." Others tell of tensions between so-called breeds and bloods not only within their families, but within the reservation community at large. In her recurrent commentary about these tensions, Becky portrays their intensity in a vivid story from her early school days:

> Their skin was lighter than mine, and they had freckles, but they talked Indian, so they considered themselves full-bloods. This one girl didn't like me, because I slapped her sister. And you know how they have those little tubs, like bird feeders or—what do you call them?—bird baths? A long time ago they used to be round, and they used to wash up in them at the boarding schools. I had my feet in there, when she came over. She called me a white woman; I had braids on and she said, "How come you have braids?" I said, "I don't know, 'cause my mom wants me to, I guess." And she said, "Well, white people don't have braids, they have short hair." And she took a scissors and she cut my braid off, right at the ear. And I just remember, she cut it and she threw it in the water. So the violence was already instilled there. All of that hatred, you know, that hatred towards the white man.

In these stories, the non-Native world figures as a powerful agent in Cheyenne lives, inspiring emotions as intense as "hatred" and motivating associated actions.

Yet while some younger women's accounts emphasize themes of the disruptive, negative impacts of the non-Native world on their developing sense of self, others cast this world as a positive resource for seeing alternatives to troubling experiences on the reservation. As such, younger women's narratives demonstrate a marked ambivalence about how the Cheyenne world is embedded within a non-Native world, and they construct a more fluid moral boundary between the two.

For example, many younger women explicitly describe how their behavior and sense of self were affected by experiences in boarding schools that produced intense feelings of fear, anger, and shame. Carol describes:

> A lot of people were abused really bad, even sexually abused. I went to boarding school, and it was really bad—we were constantly being beaten up, we couldn't speak our language, the boys and girls were kept separate and couldn't even look at each other, we had to eat certain foods all the time. It was awful. In our Cheyenne way, parents are not supposed to hit children. If you do, it makes the good spirits go away from that child. So it was shocking, to see kids being hit. The first time I saw it, I thought maybe it was an accident or something! But it wasn't.

Carol raises a number of themes here—physical and sexual abuse, suppression of language, the imposition of foreign customs regarding childhood gender relations and food choices, and violation of valued relationships with other-than-human persons. Echoing older women's accounts, her version of "our Cheyenne way" emphasizes the avoidance of physical violence in disciplining children. Yet, as she describes, witnessing these violations was "awful" and "shocking"—emotionally evocative language that was limited in older women's accounts of their negative school experiences.

Other younger women's narratives elaborate upon these themes. Echoing older women like Mary, Pauline notes the role of poverty in bringing Cheyenne children to the boarding school—but unlike older women, she also describes how the violence that she witnessed there affected her: "I remember if the boys got in a fight, the school was made out of this wall that was really hard and rough. If the boys fought, they used to have to hit that wall, even until their knuckles bled. And I thought that was pretty bad." Becky offers an especially detailed account of the emotional consequences of being raised in a rigid and punitive environment:

> I think back and I compare it to a four-year-old going into the Army. . . . And the Catholic institution, at that time, was real rigid. I was stuck there and I had to convert or be punished, and that was a real painful thing for me. . . . When I was in the fifth grade, I had to kneel

on a broomstick for two hours in front of the class, because I had a "bad attitude." I slanted my eyes and put my nose up at the Sister, so she made me do this. It was very humiliating and degrading. And I was always repenting, you know; I could have been a nun by the time I was in second grade for how much time I spent in the church repenting, so to speak, for my "unholiness!" [laughs]

Becky has devoted a lot of attention to what she wryly calls being a "recovering Catholic," as we shall see. But alongside her humor she clearly conveys the emotional climate of fear, pain, and humiliation that characterized her time at boarding school. Lynn characterizes the impact of such a climate on her childhood development: "I was in constant fear all the time being in school, and when you're in fear like that you can't open yourself up to learning."

In keeping with this portrait of the power and impact of the non-Native world on their developing selves, younger women offer more detailed accounts than older women about facing the reality that their identities as Cheyennes were stigmatized by non-Native individuals and institutions. Some comments demonstrate their childhood awareness that other features of reservation life were looked down upon by the non-Native world, and the feelings of shame that could result. Louise recalls poverty as one:

We used to camp down by the river. And these old stores and cafés used to bring like their rotten produce down to the camp. There was still some good stuff in there. It wasn't all rotten and maybe it wasn't good enough for the store anymore, but [we could use it]. And we used to, like, eat turtle, and eat dog. I think now, people are ashamed to admit [that they ate these things], but I'm not, because that was our way then.

Louise asserts her own personal lack of shame in reaction to these experiences here, but her statements clearly communicate a perception that shame is associated with such experiences and practices in the community at large.[1]

Overall, younger women's narratives emphasize how contact with the world beyond the reservation, and the cultural dynamics that it set in motion within the Northern Cheyenne community, did wield significant influence over their feelings and behavior as children. The threats posed to Cheyenne life by the surrounding non-Native world were not managed in their early lives but fundamentally altered their experience of self. Moreover, many younger women's narratives stress how, in their experiences, punitive, intimidating, and violent practices disrupted the usual course of becoming a person. In their accounts, the production of fear itself serves as a marker of undesirable and unhealthful climate for personal development. While older women frame knowledge of specific teachings as essential to their developing personhood as children, younger women articulate a somewhat different ethnopsychology that emphasizes the need for a positive emotional climate.

Yet, in addition to the accounts above, younger women are also far more likely than older women to describe non-Natives as positive resources in their lives. Despite the explicit stories of abuse, there is not a total consensus among younger women that boarding school was bad. Some women emphasize how they learned discipline and other basic positive values in boarding schools. Some also present their lives at school as a better alternative to their lives at home. Theresa remarks: "I liked it [at boarding school]. I had a bed for myself, and it was clean and I could eat, you know, three meals a day, and it was a warm place for me to be, and I made friends. So I enjoyed it over there, kind of being away from the alcoholic life of my parents." A number of community members made similar comments to me, both in interviews and in general daily social interactions. Some acknowledged experiences of violence but excused them, saying that it was still important to recognize the positive, in statements such as, "We were beaten, but we also got good education." With people that I knew well, I sometimes probed further: "But what do you think of the fact that non-Native children at that time, going to school outside of reservations, were getting a good education *without* getting beaten?" Responses varied widely. A number of people simply did not seem to want to dwell on these unpleasant features of a past era. Yet others explicitly drew links between these experiences and current problems, with one recent tribal president even initiating a lawsuit against the local Catholic boarding school for its history of exploiting and abusing Cheyenne children. Many community members expressed considerable ambivalence about the motives and wisdom of pursuing such a legal case, however, reflecting again the diversity of perceptions and interpretations of contemporary community problems on the reservation and the complex politics that often accompany efforts to respond to them.

Younger women also describe other ways in which non-Native friends and settings were positive resources in their childhood and young adult lives. In talking about her first pregnancy in late adolescence, Theresa recalls a non-Native friend who helped her considerably: "I had a real special friend at that time. She worked with 4-H. She was a white woman, and all the Indian children would go to her house, and we would cook. She taught us how to cook, sew, and all that stuff, and we'd just hang around her house, and she'd always, you know, have something for us to do, some kind of activity. And then I got to be real good friends with her." Theresa goes on to describe how this woman helped her in times of need, when her parents and siblings were not available or did not have the resources.

Alice also describes the non-Native world as an essential resource as she navigated through experiences of intense and extended sexual abuse in her childhood home. She portrays the non-Native world as a source of relief: "[When I moved off the reservation] I could really finally see that the things that were happening weren't normal and that there was a way out. It was kind of like another door opening for me."

This array of positive and negative themes often coalesce in a single narrative. For example, Becky describes the non-Native world as both a welcome alternative and an alienating one as she became more familiar with the non-Native town of Ashland while attending boarding school there:

So I started getting the idea of what life was like in the white world. And that attracted me. You know there was no drinking in the places that I was at, and people had swing sets—the modern things in life, you know, 'cause we didn't have no electricity. We made our own toys. I remember when we were growing up we had only one bicycle, everybody used it. And that attracted me. . . . Out here [in the white world], I could be safe. But I was also real isolated.

Becky clearly describes here how she linked material poverty and drinking to being Native and to being from the reservation. She also emphasizes that although the non-Native world was attractive, it was also foreign and resulted in her feeling alone and disconnected.

In sum, younger women's narratives of childhood portray the world beyond the reservation with far more ambivalence than older women's accounts. Their narratives blur the essentializing lines between Native and non-Native that are characteristic of the prominent local rhetorical conventions on the reservation and that permeate older women's accounts.

They do not attribute universally greater moral value to the Cheyenne as opposed to the non-Native worlds that they experienced as children, conveying instead that both the non-Native and Cheyenne worlds include sources of pain as well as useful resources.

Generation, Gender, and Subjectivity: Local Conversations

In describing coming of age, both older and younger women's narratives affirm how marked changes in reservation life were taking place circa 1950. Each generation's childhoods took place under very different sets of conditions, and women's narratives particularly emphasize rising economic difficulties, language loss, and domestic violence, along with a marked increase in alcohol use. Women in each generation tend to offer very different representations of the emotional dimensions of these experiences. Engaging terms and concepts from Twelve Step approaches to recovery, younger women offer detailed discussions of the emotional impact of alcohol-related neglect, abuse, and violence on their developing selves. They position alcohol use, especially by their caregivers, as a central cause of these problems. Older women describe Cheyenne personhood in terms of calm comportment, ethics of generosity and collaboration, and proper ritual conduct. They cast knowledge gained by adults teaching and children listening as essential for its development. Alcohol figures prominently in the midcentury changes that older women describe, but ultimately their narratives seem to focus primarily on the loss of Cheyenne personhood. Whether this is a cause or an effect of alcohol's rise remains an open question.

Local definitions that construct Cheyenne personhood as beyond the reach of those raised without the proper teachings are closely linked with broader rhetorical conventions that invest higher moral value in the past than the present. These discourses position many people raised under the conditions of reservation life after 1950 as deficient. Younger women's accounts demonstrate both the emotional pain and the social disenfranchisement that such positioning can produce but also incorporate Twelve Step terms and concepts to make the point that adult teachings were simply not available to them in childhood. Their narratives emphasize that they did not receive adequate instruction and teaching due to their caretakers' drinking or distraction.

The generally greater appeal of Twelve Step rhetoric to younger versus older women may in part reflect younger women's greater needs and desires to articulate these experiences, whether for emotional catharsis or to contest the social marginalization that locally dominant discourses impose. As will become clear shortly, many younger women describe sobriety itself, and the associated knowledge about a healthy emotional life, in terms of becoming a person. Casting Cheyenne personhood as achievable in sobriety rather than either fulfilled or lost in childhood offers a radical departure from prominent local constructions of personhood on the reservation.

Patterned differences in experience by generation are accompanied by distinctive rhetorical tools for representing experience, and reflect different models of fundamental cultural concepts such as personhood. As such, the diversity of perspectives on alcohol and pathways toward sobriety among Northern Cheyenne women has significant psychological depth, grounded in different subjectivities that have in turn been shaped by the changing historical conditions of reservation life.

Yet younger women's discussions of their childhood lives also hint at the limits of a conventional Twelve Step framework for accounting for historical experiences that impact personhood in Northern Cheyenne and other Native American communities, such as the specifics of language loss and forced-assimilation approaches in boarding schools. A model of "alcoholic" family dynamics does not fully account for how local cultural identity is uniquely at stake for Northern Cheyenne community members, or for how the "teachings" that produce Cheyenne persons are not simply about being an adult but also include additional goals of maintaining cultural difference and managing dispossession within a racialized social order. An awareness of these historical processes also informs younger women's constructions of Cheyenne personhood as disrupted rather than irrevocably lost.

For example, Jenny describes her grandfather's experiences with institutions such as boarding schools, a cornerstone of policies of forced assimilation in the early twentieth century, and how she and her siblings did not listen when he advised them not to drink.

> He was sent to a boarding school when he was really young . . . and there was a time when they . . . shamed them for being Indian, and that's when the white man was trying to take away . . . all of the Indianness out of these old people. And so after that he just became a Christian, but he would always tell us . . . that alcohol is bad for you and smoking is bad for you and that [he] quit smoking and drinking

when [he] was 18. . . . But we didn't listen. We had all the answers, or we thought that we did.

Jenny portrays her grandfather as having lost important elements that she values in being Cheyenne, such as spirituality and pride in cultural distinctiveness from the dominant society. While here she chides herself and her siblings for not listening to him, she also conveys their sense that his authority was undermined in their eyes by his own identity confusion. Jenny therefore advances a historicized account of how the psychological sequellae of colonization came to be passed from previous generations to her own.

Comparative analysis of women's stories of their lives as they reached adulthood and pursued sobriety, the topics of the next two chapters, further illuminates these themes and their interplay in local community life at Northern Cheyenne. The ways in which women's experiences of gender both compare and contrast by generation, addressed briefly here in discussions of gender roles and especially gender-based violence in childhood, become clearer particularly in women's accounts of their relationships with partners and spouses in adulthood.

5
Family Lives and Gendered Experience

Women's narratives of reaching adulthood illuminate how they variably construct their social roles as adult women, and their understandings of how alcohol use by themselves and others impact the fulfillment of those roles. Older and younger Northern Cheyenne women offer similar portraits of forming families under conditions of widespread drinking on the reservation. In particular, both focus centrally on experiences and concerns that surround their roles as adult members of their natal kin groups, as spouses/partners forming new households (for those who have done so), and as caregivers to children. Caregivers on the reservation are commonly mothers, but many older- and younger-generation women also play primary caregiving roles to children as grandmothers, aunts, and so forth. The extensive local history of collective approaches to child rearing seems visible here, yet these practices also stem from current realities in which it is not uncommon for women's own children and/or siblings to be unable to fulfill their caregiving roles for reasons as varied as work responsibilities, educational pursuits, and involvement in drinking.

Central problems that both older and younger women emphasize in their accounts of adulthood, whether in their own lives or in observations of other community members, include tense social relationships with natal kin, discord and violence in relationships with intimate partners, and the abuse and neglect of children. This commentary attests to a broadly shared investment in local standards of caregiving among Northern Cheyenne women across generations, and related concerns about threats to household functioning and to child rearing. Women also broadly share in associated social commentary about the impact of changing gender roles on family life, which often takes the form of critiques of men's changing roles and behavior.

Yet, despite these similarities, profound differences are also evident in how members of each generational group discuss these topics. These differences further illustrate the workings of distinctive ethnopsychologies of Cheyenne personhood in women's commentary and illuminate the gendered dimensions of how women use both local rhetorical tools and those drawn from Twelve Step approaches to recovery.

Older Women: Witnessing Pervasive Disruption

In keeping with their narratives of childhood, older women's narratives emphasize how the development of persons has been fundamentally altered on the reservation, such that Northern Cheyenne community members are increasingly oriented around new and negative values and practices. In a recurrent idiom with clear echoes of Sweet Medicine's prophecies, older women describe people "forgetting" the lessons of childhood. More clearly here than in their narratives of childhood, older women also describe the use of alcohol in terms of "forgetting" how one was taught to behave, and they position drinking as a symptom rather than a cause of this wide-ranging process of moral loss.

While describing some continuities with valued elements of childhood, older women's accounts of their adult lives generally portray how conflict, disrespect, and dissolution had replaced earlier standards of comportment and affect. They portray the moral erosion that began in later childhood or adolescence as intensifying in their adult lives. Kinship and ritual resources that previously helped to manage threats to well-being among tribal members sustained damage, and core values and ethics such as generosity and collaboration have been "forgotten" and replaced by widespread self-focus and greed in reservation life.

For example, older women's stories of their experiences in forming households and raising children are infused with generalized statements contrasting "people today" with those of the past. While this rhetoric is also evident in their narratives of childhood, older women's accounts of adulthood further emphasize how those who "know" how to be appropriate Cheyenne persons experience increasing isolation on the reservation. Younger generations figure prominently in these accounts as lacking the knowledge needed to think, feel, and behave appropriately.

Many of these comments are cast in very general terms, such as Sara's: "We were taught to walk away from a fight. That's something that people have really forgotten today." Here, generalized "people" have forgotten the lessons of proper comportment that she learned in childhood and have moved from valuing a calm and even-tempered demeanor to recurrently participating in social discord.

Some women's commentary included not just behavior, but imputed motives. As Rosemary remarked about local politics: "Nowadays they need 20 people for a quorum at a district meeting—and they never have it. No one comes. People are only interested in money or gossip." "Gossip" here refers not simply to discussion of other people, but to negative talk intended to malign a person's reputation and standing. Such talk contradicts the conflict-reducing comportment that older women's accounts privilege. Northern Cheyenne "people" are now oriented by values and priorities that concern power politics and material gain, rather than collective good. Older women's comments about conflicts among local ritual leaders include similar themes. Laura remarks that the ethos of circumspection, modesty, and restraint that characterized such pursuits in her early life had changed: "My dad didn't want to be called a medicine man, or head man—it was too high. There was something real special about it. In them days you had to earn it. Now they call people medicine men that are too young. I wonder where they learned it, and I never seen them earn it." She emphasizes here that the dedication and difficulty of these ritual roles are now overlooked in favor of desires for attention and recognition. Some explicitly link contemporary community problems to corruption of ritual protocol. Laura elaborates, "In my father's day he was real careful [in following ceremonial protocol], and there were no wrecks or people shooting themselves." Other women specifically reference interpersonal conflict among ceremonial people, as a source of further social discord. At the time that I conducted many life history interviews, a serious controversy over the Sacred Buffalo Hat during the past year was still fresh in many women's minds. Rosemary observes: "Things were more peaceful, in my time. The [Sacred Buffalo Hat] Bundle was taken care of; there was no fighting." Such comments convey that what had helped to sustain the Northern Cheyenne world of their early lives is now threatened by the encroachment of negative values and conflict-promoting behaviors.

Themes of decline are similarly evident in older women's accounts of Christian churches, which along with Cheyenne ritual practices had also helped to enact and perpetuate collaborative social relations in their childhood lives. For example, Laura notes how by her adulthood, her church had essentially "fallen apart": "I used to teach Bible school, and here my grandchildren don't even know anything about Bible school. By the time I got married, the church seemed to be falling apart. Women would get mad at each other, gossip. The pastors were fighting with each other. Driving people away." Here, Laura specifically emphasizes how concern with power plays overwhelmed appropriate concern for the well-being of the church itself or of congregation members.

Older women widely implicate a similar moral decline as a cause of trouble in other prominent local institutions. Again using the broad rhetoric of "people," Rosemary speaks critically of the emergence of greed in tribal government: "People spend money like water. The Tribal Council . . . had to cut down [payments to council members per meeting] since they got in the red so much. My brother used to be on the council, when they got $5 per meeting. At that time they did per cap [per capita] payments and really helped their people; they were in there for the people, not the money."

Older women commonly describe feelings of isolation and loss upon witnessing these changes. Sara repeatedly emphasizes how these changes amount to a loss of respect and caring, noting, for example, "I visited one of those brand new houses in Lame Deer, and it was just messy—clothes everywhere, food everywhere. They don't care anymore." Sara describes how these widespread patterns of disrespect have impacted her sense of self and connection to other women of her own generation:

> There was still a lot of respect in my day—like my husband, I respect him. I don't go do what I want—I ask him, respect his opinion. Maybe the change came after my day. I do notice—I was taught that you never tease your brother or [male] cousin, or say anything bad to them. And I see that a lot of times with women my age. Like they'll tease them in a dirty, nasty way and then laugh. I just sit there. I sit there and think, "I must be the only one who still believes that way." They really are losing respect, come to think of it. They don't care what they say.

"I sit there and think, 'I must be the only one'" is a significant statement of altered subjectivity compared to earlier eras of life, a move from feelings of connection to a sense of isolation. While painting a broad portrait of "people" and clearly including members of their own generation, many older women especially focus on the negative values and improper behaviors of younger generations.

The bulk of older women's narratives of adulthood, however, focused on the negative values and disruptive behaviors that played out in their own personal experiences in roles as kin/family members, spouses/partners, and caregivers to children. The most intense expressions of emotion by older women during the interviews took place when they discussed losses of or serious troubles in relations with close kin.

Natal Kinship: Unraveling Ties

Older women's narratives overwhelmingly emphasize the loss of collaborative kin relations that were formed with siblings, cousins, and others in their earlier lives, whether through premature death or through social conflict. They recurrently link alcohol to these losses but variously foreground and background its causal role.

Many women describe how they simply lost family members to alcohol-related violence, including stabbings, shootings, and car wrecks. Their accounts emphasize how such events produced considerable emotional pain, such as from the shock associated with the unexpectedness of the death, finding or having to go identify the body, and having to come to terms with the nature or degree of violence involved. Women also describe feeling overwhelmed by the sheer frequency of alcohol-related deaths. Among the women that I interviewed, it is common to have lost at least one if not more immediate relatives to alcohol-related violence. Several also emphasize the stress of having to continue living in a relatively small community that includes the person or people responsible for their loved one's death (and who, depending on the vagaries of the federal, state, and/or tribal legal systems, might or might not have been penalized).

Beyond the outright severing of relationships through loss, older women often also describe their adult relations with surviving kin as strained. Themes of smoldering conflict and/or distance in their relationships with siblings are common, such as Ruth's example of a troubled relationship with her brother.

> My father died of metastatic cancer. He was getting worse and worse. I took him to clinic, and that's where they could see that it had spread. My brother blamed me for taking him to clinic—like that was what made [him] get so sick. Then when my mother got sick, my brother wanted her in a nursing home. I wanted to take care of her at home, so I did. My brother was mad. Then later he was having trouble with his marriage, and I gave him advice. He didn't like what I said. He has

not spoken to me since and told his kids not to speak to me, either. It's been about eight years now.

Such intense ongoing tensions clearly undermine the capacity for aunts and uncles to play roles in the daily lives of their nephews and nieces.

Conflicts with siblings and cousins were also frequently noted and discussed in daily life on the reservation during my residence there. One friend witnessed a flare in a long-smoldering conflict between two older women who were close relatives, at a family social event. The elder of the two initiated a verbal confrontation about events that had happened several decades earlier, and the exchange was so tense that the whole gathering went quiet for several minutes. As the other woman left, the elder woman subsequently commented to my friend: "I don't want her in my house, I don't want her calling me up. The only time she comes over here is when she wants something." This statement contrasts starkly with the collective, cooperative ethos in older women's accounts of family life in their childhoods, characterizing the relationship in terms of abuse and exploitation rather than reciprocity and collaboration. The speaker specifically charges the other woman with self-focused greed ("wants something"). Like Ruth's above, this story also attests to the intense and protracted social tension that can accompany emotionally intense family conflicts.

Older women do not usually explicitly position alcohol as a component of these stories, even though it often seems to have been present in the lives of those involved. By not offering this or another specific causal explanation, these stories imply that trouble emerges from the participants themselves: Cheyennes have become fundamentally different sorts of people, in their motives and actions, compared to the past. Articulating similar themes, older women's narratives of their adult lives heavily focus upon problems with forming new households and families. These accounts especially feature commentary about changing gender roles and relations.

Married Life: The Decline of Male Social Roles

Older women's stories of getting married and starting families include considerable criticism of changes in men's behaviors and roles, and highlight how local rhetorical conventions for comparing past with present can have gendered dimensions. Motifs of interpersonal tension pervade many of their portraits of relationships with husbands. Yet, while prominent, these themes are not universal. Some older women do por-tray their marriages as workable partnerships, and as desired. Sara says: "I had big plans as a girl. I went to college, and the church paid for my tuition. But then I met my husband, and I forgot all about school! [laughs] We knew pretty soon that we wanted to get married." Sara describes her-self as marrying for love, and she offers a number of stories of positive interactions with her husband—for example, how they would tease each other, and how they generally seemed have a companionable and mutu-ally supportive relationship.

Moore (1999) asserts that Cheyenne marriages do not tend to be structured around the kind of romantic love that is so culturally elabo-rated within the United States. Rather, affection and regard develop over time in marriages that last. Yet, while I found that standards of attention, affection, and respect that are broadly similar to mainstream U.S. cul-tural conceptions of love were more common among younger than older women, these did figure in some older women's accounts of their experi-ences and expectations of marriage. While it is certainly likely that a con-cept of romantic love or some modified form of it has gained currency at Northern Cheyenne relatively recently, pre–reservation era stories of young women committing suicide at the loss of their betrothed in battle (e.g., Grinnell 1972a) do seem to attest to the presence of some notions of romantic attachment to a particular individual in Cheyenne cultural history. Nonetheless, generational contrasts in commentary about mari-tal relationships are also evident, as I witnessed during one recent sum-mer visit to the reservation following the breakup of a younger-genera-tion woman's long-term marriage. Younger women tended to support the wife's decision to end the marriage due to the husband's recurrent infidelity, which left her feeling humiliated and angry and unable to trust him. Older women tended to emphasize how the husband had fulfilled his economic role as provider to her family, however, and to express how the occasional indiscretions of a man who "works hard every day" should be overlooked. Indeed, as older women described negative expe-riences of marriage during the interviews, they overwhelmingly empha-sized male failures to fulfill the roles of provider and protector rather than ideals of emotional attachment.

A number of older women express marked ambivalence in recalling how and why they entered into marriage. Josephine describes with char-acteristic humor how she came to marry a troubled and troubling man, not from attraction so much as from a sense of limited options, since her primary caregivers had died when she was still in her teens: "I think the reason why I got married right away is because I really didn't have no place to stay in Ashland. I really—that was just my escape, or . . . I don't know. I always say, why did I rush into it, you know, I could have . . . I could have just stayed at Mission. Maybe by now I'll be a Sister! [laughs]"

Many older women's narratives of marriage and family life are interwoven with more general comments on negative changes in male roles, and prominent local rhetorical conventions of relating past to present are visible in how they use men from their childhood lives as points of comparison. Vicky comments: "In those days, men were more involved in planting, working. Now they're just lazy—you don't see them plant, except maybe a few. And a lot of them don't even work—maybe just once in a while."

A key theme throughout this commentary is the greater involvement of Northern Cheyenne women in economic roles outside of the home, relative to their parents' generation. Nearly all of the older women that I interviewed emphasized the decline of men's roles as economic providers by their adult lives. This change seems to have met with a number of contradictory responses. Some women describe work outside the home as a source of pride and enjoyment (e.g., taking on supervisory positions, receiving training, traveling to workshops), and/or as an extension of their role as caretakers in the family (see also Moore 1999; Ward et al. 1995). Yet as Straus (1976) records, in the early 1970s many Northern Cheyenne community members viewed women working outside the home as a sign that times were very bad for a family. An assumption that the man should support the family is clearly at work here, and in my own fieldwork, decades later, the notion that women had to work because men were failing to fulfill their provider roles was recurrently emphasized in the narratives of older women.

Many older women describe how their own efforts at employment outside the home became a source of tension in their marriages. Esther remarks: "I couldn't please him or do anything right. He was very hard to live with. He tried to stop me from working, but I insisted on going. He had no job. I always worked, even when I was pregnant. I wanted to feed my children." Here, Esther conveys her own sense that someone needed to work to provide for the children, and that her husband did not recognize or share this priority. Instead of fulfilling his gender-specific responsibility as a provider, he focused instead on trying to control her.

Jealous accusations about suspected infidelity figure prominently in women's descriptions of marital tensions associated with their employment. Laura describes how jealousy shaped her husband's expressions of discomfort with her working: "My husband was jealous of me if I was working. He would accuse me like I was sneaking around behind his back, seeing other men. I quit jobs because of his accusations."

Both Esther and Laura also reference drinking as a component of their husband's behavior. Yet neither clearly position alcohol as a cause of men's lack of employment or negative reactions to their wives' employment. Instead, most older women's accounts focus more on the proximate scope of alcohol-related behaviors by their husbands. For example, Mary describes how her own drinking was mild, and it was her husband's drinking and violence that caused problems in the family: "I tried it but it didn't agree with me. When I first met my husband, I would drink a beer here and there. Any more than one or two, and I would throw up, get sick. So after about 10 years, I quit it. I started to hate it. Alcohol really affected my husband. He would hit me, and the kids would see. He was really mean. We would go stay someplace else until he sobered up." She clearly links her husband's "mean" and violent behavior to the times during which he was drinking, and uses the strong term "hate" to describe the intense negative emotions that she experienced in response to the disrespect of his violent behavior. The central importance that she places on raising children is also clear in how she frames the damage of her husband's violence as being worst when the children witnessed it.

Here again, Josephine departs somewhat from other older women's styles of describing male behavior by offering a more detailed psychological explanation, attributing her husband's behavior to his continuing dependency on his mother: "It was like, he didn't want to stay away from the old place, you know. He was afraid, afraid to have a home. Because over there, you know, his mom furnished everything. Like if we ran out of food, he'd say, 'Well, I'll go to mom's and get that. I'll go to mom's.' And it would be different if he'd said, 'Well, let me go see if I can find a job.'" She portrays her husband as fundamentally unwilling to take on the responsibility of a new household and family. His personal development, in her view, had simply not led him to be oriented to or invested in a role as provider.

Despite its more psychological dimension, however, Josephine's account is similar to other older women's in providing an experiential perspective on the lack of autonomy and dependability that she encountered in her marriage partner. Such perspectives focus not on the economic conditions of reservation life and the challenges that Northern Cheyenne men face in fulfilling the provider role in this environment, but instead on the immediate relationship dynamics that the speaker experienced.

Many older women go on to describe how these marital dynamics affected their own alcohol consumption. Mary's husband's drinking ultimately led *her* to quit drinking. But many other older women describe how establishing a new household with a man who drank actually led them, at least at first, to intensify their own drinking.

Drinking Careers: "You Don't Know What You're Doing"

When discussing their own use of alcohol, older women emphasize how they violated moral values learned (and experienced) in childhood, a form of their own "forgetting." While women's accounts vary, they frequently focus on the impact of their drinking upon family formation, marriage, and child rearing. This thematic emphasis suggests that older women prioritize these gender-specific social roles.

Many describe how their husbands influenced them to drink more, and how their escalating alcohol use worked to intensify problems of economic strain and household tension. Laura recounts:

> Then I got married, and my husband liked to drink. He had a lot of friends. I didn't drink as much, because I had little ones to look after. When my kids grew up, I would go to town with them and my sisters and drink beer. Sometimes my mom and dad would tell me to leave the kids, and not take them; so I would leave the older ones to take care of themselves. We would get beer and drive all over. I lost three good jobs from drinking. I was bumming money from my folks, sisters, friends. I would say I'd pay them back, but I had no job. I would drink around, sit at Jimtown [a local off-reservation bar] with my husband until someone would offer us a drink. We were living on G.A. [general assistance, a public assistance program administered by the B.I.A.] once in a while. I hocked stuff, to buy drinks.

Laura's emphasis on caring for children is noteworthy as a statement of gender-specific responsibilities. But Laura also links her drinking with transgressing these responsibilities, as well as others, for example, "bumming" from family and friends rather than fulfilling reciprocal obligations. She portrays her social functioning as having gone broadly astray here.

Josephine offers a similarly structured narrative but emphasizes how her husband's use of brute force played a role: "He used to drink a lot. And pretty soon we started having kids, and things started going wrong because he would drink. He would start beating me up. I think that's when he really forced me to drink. Boy, he would just pour wine all over me, beat me up. So, I started drinking with him. I started drinking so I wouldn't feel the pain. But [then] I really got into alcohol, too." Her story continues with marked similarities to Laura's account of how drinking undermined her capacity to keep a job, and promoted pawning and selling to get money for alcohol.

> Boy, a lot of things happened, you know. Oh shoot I had fun, I thought it was fun. But there were lot of things that happened. I got to the point where I would drink on weekends, like two days, and then a time came when it kind of got out of control. I stayed out of work for about three days, like my friend said, "Well, here, drink this and you'll make it through the day." You know, take a drink and I'd go to work? Stuff like that. And then pretty soon, I'd go home, save some, hide some wine, drink at noon and some evenings. And then pretty soon, I didn't go back to work. I got fired. Boy, I was really drinking. Even if I didn't have any money, somebody would come around. Or you just go down to Jimtown, they'd say, "Oh, you want a drink?" Or, go hock something, or sell something.

While these accounts emphasize how men's drinking influences women's, older women did not describe alcohol's effects in their marriages as unilateral. Laura emphasizes female as well as male responsibility for these consequences, for example, in speaking of the bad feelings and conflict that alcohol can inspire.

> When you're drunk, you don't know what you're saying or doing. I would fight with my husband, we would argue, accuse each other ("you were with that man" or "you were with that woman"). Remember bad things from the past, and bring them up. Maybe that's how alcohol works. Push each other, call each other names ("the hell with you" and "shut up"). Say, "I'm leaving tomorrow and I don't want to see you." Forget what you're really talking about. Then sober up, feel real

sorry—can't even remember what you said or why. Those are bad feelings—you don't mean what you said, but you already said it.

Here again, the idiom of "forgetting" appears in a description of alcohol-related behavior. Laura's narrative also emphasizes the careless and destructive features of alcohol-related interactions, a clear contrast with the emphasis on careful speech and respect for the power of language that she and many other older women highlighted as a key childhood teaching.

Ultimately, like other older women who came to sobriety, Laura describes how she came to desire a stable job and to resent the impact of household violence on herself and her kids. She portrays how her husband, however, continued to make jealous accusations, drink, and initiate physical conflicts rather than contribute constructively to the household.

But then I told him I would apply and keep a job, and I did it. He didn't like it. I was working with a man, and my husband called him "your new boyfriend." I said, "I won't listen to you." He went out and drank, and came back to raise hell. He hit me, and I hit him. I got a restraining order, everything. I moved his clothes out. I was tired of him. He wasn't helping me, the kids were scared of him. I got a divorce.

Now moving in a fundamentally different direction from her husband, Laura took action to end her marriage. She portrays this response as very determined, going so far as to make use of local institutions such as law enforcement to implement a restraining order. While some older women do not report such negative experiences with husbands who drank, and others describe weathering household problems until their husbands reached a point where they found their own compelling reasons to limit or entirely quit drinking, a number of other older women echo Laura's portrait of how unhappiness with their economic situations and family lives during their drinking years ultimately contributed to decisions to divorce.

The impact of this greater family instability and the general community climate on children is apparent in older women's accounts of parenthood. As with their discussions of men's roles, however, these accounts often do not articulate specific causes or describe alcohol as an especially central factor in these troubling new realities.

Raising Children in Changing Times: Younger Generations in Decline

Older women's stories of the challenges of raising children emphasize the difficulty of serving as caregivers in an environment that includes multiple negative influences on personal behavior and development. While they clearly position drinking and drug use among these negative influences, their narratives often position substance use as only one element in a broader process of collective moral decline.

Older women frequently tell stories about the decline of sexual regulation in their children's lives. As a key example, they highlight the rise of unexpected and out-of-wedlock pregnancies in recent decades. Mary recounts: "My daughter got in trouble when she was a teenager. Her boyfriend was older, and gave her drinks." This description places the responsibility on the male and directly implicates alcohol. But many women also note how sexual mores on the reservation have changed for both females and males. Anne remarks: "Now, if girls have a boyfriend, they'll be with them every day, even stay at their house. And girls go to pick boys up—before, boys would come to the house. Well, we never had cars, anyway! But the women and girls today are just more aggressive." Such statements again imply fundamental changes in the types and qualities of people who constitute the community.

Many older women do mention their attempt to pass on the same teachings to their children that they had learned in childhood about the dangers of alcohol and sexual assault. Martha notes, "I used to tell my daughter that too, 'Don't be alone with your dad or your brothers if they're drinking—they don't know what they're doing. Go stay with your aunt or your grandma if I'm not here. Stay away from any man that's drinking.'" Here, Martha seems to be playing the same role as her own mother and grandmother, in warning her to stay away from men that are drinking. At the same time, though, she tells her daughter to seek out female supervision on her own—an explicit departure from the "back then, someone was always watching you" themes of older women's narratives about their early lives. Martha also directly implicates her husband as a potential abuser, an attribution that did not appear in older generations' discussions of their own fathers or of their mother's advice. Here again, then, disordered sexual and gender relations figure as a key site for older women's depictions of witnessing moral decline from their early to later lives.

Older women also report witnessing a rise in domestic violence in their children's lives, compared to their own. While some experienced violence in their own marriages, Sara did not. She describes her intense shock when she learned that her son was drinking heavily and hitting his wife, and her feelings of frustration when his behavior persisted despite her efforts to talk with him. While drinking is clearly involved in this story, Sara does not explicitly portray alcohol as the cause of her son's behavior. Her account implies instead that the context of community life has changed for the worse and influences her son more than either his experiences growing up in her household or her efforts to advise him.

Josephine also describes her children's behavior in terms of decline. Her complex combination of affirming and departing from key themes in other older women's narratives also appears in her account of how her drinking affected her children. She differs from other older women in explicitly implicating her own drinking in her children's subsequent alcohol use. This idea is encapsulated in the Twelve Step notion of "cycles," familiar to Josephine from her extensive involvement in recovery activities on the reservation. She describes that although she did not drink with her kids directly, her alcohol use clearly set an example for them and disrupted her relationships with them.

> It started hurting really bad when my girls started turning to alcohol. But it was so—I couldn't say anything. I was afraid, afraid to say something 'cause they'd say, "Well, mom, you done that. We learned it from you," you know. "You used to drink. And you never used to listen to us, so why should we listen to you?" you know. And I say, "Well, don't do it because I did." But that's what most of them used on me: "You did it, why shouldn't I?"

Significantly too, Josephine describes here how her drinking presented her children with grounds not only for their own drinking, but also for openly challenging her authority as a parent. Stories of such open and hostile challenges to adult authority are rare in older women's discussions of their own childhoods and further substantiate older women's general rhetorical emphasis on bearing witness to dramatic transgressions of the moral worlds that predominated in their early lives.

Josephine and other older women with the most intense drinking careers are most likely to acknowledge the impact that their drinking had on their children. But even these accounts do not clearly attribute great causal power to alcohol itself. In describing her drinking career, for instance, Laura highlights how she tried to limit the impact of her drinking on her kids by leaving them alone or with relatives. Josephine similarly remarks:

> Kids need something, and rather than use that money to get what they wanted, I'll go get drunk. Come back home and they'd say, "Well, did you get it?" you know? "Oh, I went and drank," you know. It's true, when they say kids suffer the most. But we hardly ever drank around my kids. Most of the time my sister-in-law would take them, or my mother-in-law, you know, leave 'em there—or my aunt. Maybe if I was around them all the time, maybe they would get me mad, or maybe I would hit them or slap them up, or, you know, things like that. And that's one thing I'm happy about, that I hardly ever drank around them.

Both Laura and Josephine explicitly frame accounts of their drinking practices around cultural standards of maternal behavior, marking their ongoing awareness of these standards even when they consumed alcohol heavily. In these ways, both rhetorically limit alcohol's power to disrupt their roles as mothers, therefore implying that factors beyond drinking are responsible for growing disruptions of women's caregiving roles in other households on the reservation.

Whether they point to influences inside or outside of natal households, all older women emphasize that their children's generation has become even more involved in drinking and drug use than their own had. Mary observes, "There's more drinking today than when we were growing up," while Sara elaborates: "There are more young people drinking than there used to be. It still bothers me to see young people smoking in front of their parents, too. That would never happen, in my day." Some specifically stress how children became distracted by alcohol and drugs and no longer listened to their parents.[1] Vicky tells of how she saw her kids and stepkids adopt a lifestyle of substance use that included getting married, getting divorced, and not working consistently. "They haven't done anything with their lives," she concludes.

For many older women, these comments figure in a larger portrait of moral erosion with multiple causes and manifestations that extend beyond alcohol. Many point to wider-ranging disruptions in the transmission of cultural knowledge to younger generations, for example. As Sara comments: "Young people don't even know who they're related to anymore. Maybe that's why having no respect has gotten so out of hand. All of these break-ins. The other day, my sister said that someone stole her gas [out of her car's gas tank]. She said, 'I suppose it's one of my grandkids, anyway!'" Sara also emphasizes how she witnessed the decline of Cheyenne language in her children's and grandchildren's generations, as well as in the community at large.

> My grandpa used to tell us a lot of stories—Indian fairy tales. I wrote them all down. I tell my grandkids about them, if they're at the house at night. I write them in English, but it's not as good as when you hear it in Cheyenne. I don't even use Cheyenne when I go to the store anymore. Seems like there's not very many real old people, who don't understand English, anymore. . . . The schools are trying to teach Cheyenne, but it doesn't stay with the kids. They don't remember even a couple of days later. You got to speak it at home.

Sara describes herself as habitually thinking in Cheyenne and translating in her head before speaking, and in one conversation told me how she wanted to spare her children from having to do so, as well as from being punished for not knowing English in school. She also expressed ambivalence about how she focused on teaching her kids English, however. Over a year and a half or so, I asked her about this a couple of times. Her responses varied widely, from a catch in her voice while expressing regret on one occasion to a firm "But I would still do it again" on another. Some unresolved tension seems evident here. While Sara acknowledges the difficulty and tragedy of language loss, she also seems to not want to devote too much time and energy to regretting decisions that she had made under the pressures that she faced at the time.

While older women as a whole seem to agree that younger generations embody a decline in Cheyenne personhood, they vary in whether and how they offer explicit interpretations of exactly why. Upon closer examination, however, many of their descriptions emphasize the loss of valued Cheyenne ways of being and their replacement with destructive alternatives derived from the non-Native world.

Causes of Moral Decline: Encroaching Non-Native Values

While older women emphasize the management of threats posed by non-Native individuals and institutions in their early lives, their narratives of adulthood offer quite a different portrait. Some accounts employ a logic of exceptionalism. Mae tells how she learned to overcome her feelings of shyness and "mingle" with white people through her work as a cook, assisting with banquets and other events at one of the reservation's government schools. As an adult she went on to be active in local and regional politics from time to time, speaking out on behalf of the reservation's needs, clearly taking pride in her ability to do so and sometimes commenting that the community needs more people who are willing to take these kinds of actions. Annie describes her brother's ability to find and keep jobs that require interacting with non-Natives, contrasting him and herself to other Cheyennes "too bashful" to do so. These statements at once substantiate a general tendency among tribal members to feel intimidated by the non-Native world and, in the same motion, rhetorically stress transcending this tendency in their particular cases.

More often, though, older women explicitly implicate the encroaching of the non-Native world on the moral world of their early lives. Vicky describes change as a process of being seduced by the opportunities afforded by the non-Native world, leading to an excessive focus outside home and household. She specifically mentions the decline of gardening and other home-centered activities so characteristic of her early childhood, saying, "Now nobody don't want to stay home and do these things. They want to get into a fast life. I still enjoy cooking, and picking berries. Now people want to go to town."

Rising materialistic values and consumerism are also prominent themes in older women's critical commentary about how life "now" compared to earlier periods in their lives. For example, Mary describes how she initially adopted the definitions of wealth and poverty presented by mainstream U.S. society but later came to question their appropriateness: "[When I was a child] I thought we were really poor, because we never had candy and it was hard to buy new clothes or new shoes. But now when I think of it, we were better off—we had chickens, a milk cow, horses. We had plenty." In a similar portrait of seduction followed by correction, Vivian describes how she neglected her children in her pursuit of financial success: "I had one job, and I got a second job. I got on the fast lane, with white people—earning money, sending kids to college. I would work eight hours, spend one hour with kids, go back to work in the evening until 2 a.m. I worked when I was sick. I neglected my kids." This statement also rhetorically parallels some women's discussions, described above, of how alcohol use caused them to forgo their family responsibilities.

In these ways, older women seem to position alcohol as one element of the growing influence of the non-Native world and its values in Cheyenne life. Questions of why these changes have occurred seem far less marked in their narratives than questions about how and among whom.

Summary: Rhetorics of Moral Decline

Older women's narratives of reaching adulthood employ prominent local rhetorical conventions that define the past as a moral compass and source of expectations and values that have been violated by later experience. Kinship ties, gender roles, and language loss are among the most common sites of these violations highlighted by their accounts. Older women's discussion and displays of emotion during the interviews were strongest when telling stories of deaths in the family and disrupted kin relations, suggesting that such troubles were especially significant for them.

Older women seem to variously attribute these changes to violations of ritual protocol, the "forgetting" of childhood teachings, the seductiveness of non-Native ways, and the use of alcohol. All are mixed together in their accounts, as characterizing or contributing to the loss of Cheyenne persons that possess the knowledge and ethics needed for proper social behavior. In keeping with this rhetorical emphasis on a loss of personhood, older women express criticism for members of their own generations and for tribal government and ritual leaders but especially focus on how key forms of knowledge are systematically lacking in later generations. Younger women, in contrast, continue to draw quite different connections between age and personhood in their narratives of coming to adulthood.

Younger Women: "Cycles" of Alcoholism, Codependency, and Historical Trauma

Younger women's narratives of their lives as adults show much thematic overlap with older women's, also focusing on their roles with families and especially as spouses/partners and caregivers to children. But younger women's accounts diverge markedly from older women's in focusing on the psychological dimensions of drinking as a central cause of patterns and cycles of emotional pain, learned behavior, and social pressure that underwrite both alcohol use and unhealthy social relationships in their adult lives. Moreover, younger women describe key community institutions that could be offering assistance with these problems as unjust or nonfunctional or troubled—with reference not to alternatives from their earlier lives, but to more abstract understandings that morally proper behavior expresses one's own emotional well-being and protects that of others.

Continuing the Twelve Step framework of cycles that many employed in their narratives of childhood, many younger women's accounts of their adult lives also describe tension and difficulty in key relationships with natal kin, husbands, and children. For many too, the drinking careers that they initiated in childhood or adolescence continued into adulthood, sometimes intensifying in response to particularly stressful events.

Substance Use and Disrupted Kinship

Like older women, younger women describe variable quality in their relationships with natal family members in adulthood. Many describe conflict, but some also portray their relationships with parents and siblings as important resources in their daily lives. Jeanne mixes both themes in depicting her relationships with her siblings. Early in her narrative she emphasizes themes of "closeness" and aid: "My brothers and sisters, we're really close. You know, it's not a day goes by we don't see each other. You know, when we need help, we help each other. Or if we need money, if they have it, they'll give it to me, or if I have it, I'll give it to them, or if they need my car, you know, I'll let them use it. They say some of them, they don't really help each other that much. But we're really close." By explicitly contrasting her own close sibling relationships with others' in the community, Jeanne marks her awareness that strife and distance in families are also common. She seems to take pride in maintaining these connections during their general decline among other community members. Yet at a later point, Jeanne also expresses frustration with her siblings for drinking and smoking with her kids: "I tried to tell them too, like my older one, they used to drink with him. Or smoke. And I would try to tell them 'Don't do that to my son, that's your nephew. I wouldn't do that to your kids. I wouldn't drink with your kids, or I wouldn't offer your kids "Do you want to smoke?" or "Do you want to take this?" I would never do that,' you know." Here she emphasizes how substance use can interfere with proper kinship ties, provoking considerable tension.

Indeed, most younger women emphasize tension and conflict in their portraits of kin ties. Julie describes feeling exploited in her relationships with natal family members. "I don't really have much contact with all of [my immediate family members]. The closeness isn't there, even with my mom. If they come see me, [it] is when they want something. They want to borrow money, or they want to borrow this, or they need help with something. They want me to fix it. That's the only time I ever hear from them. They don't just come to my house and visit." At another point, Julie extends this pattern to her father: "When he comes I know something is wrong." She then relates her own efforts to come to terms with these family dynamics as part of her recovery from codependency, which involves distinguishing positive caretaking and helpfulness from exploitation and abuse.

There is a striking rhetorical similarity here to some older women's comments, which took the form of "they only come around here when they want something." Yet, despite this overlap, younger women do not juxtapose such comments against previous experiences of connection and care as older women do. It is noteworthy, too, that older women really discussed only siblings and children in this manner, while younger women such as Julie extend this commentary to intergenerational relationships, criticizing their parents and other members of older generations. References to the Twelve Step concept of codependency were also virtually absent in older women's accounts of family tension, but common in younger women's.

Marital Dynamics and the Perpetuation of "Cycles"

Younger women tend to employ a characteristically Twelve Step notion of the reproduction of "cycles" through which feelings of hurt and fear, abandonment, and shame in their childhood lives spurred a vicious cycle of unhealthy interpersonal relationships and alcohol use in adulthood, including those with spouses. For example, Jenny describes how being raised by her grandfather did not provide her with a female role model, leaving her feeling confused and empty. She began drinking as a teenager, but her use of alcohol intensified in early adulthood when she married a violent man who drank heavily, and she eventually divorced him.

In Jenny's narrative, alcohol use figures as an effort to cope with these emotionally painful situations.

Similarly, younger women's discussions of their relationships with men articulate themes of violence, alcohol, and absence similar to those of older women, yet focus far more on the psychological or emotional dynamics involved. In their frequent stories of domestic violence, younger women often portray these events as replays of what they had witnessed between their own parents. Theresa and Louise both describe their own experiences of alcohol-related marital violence in this fashion. Theresa says: "Whenever we would both drink, we'd fight each other. I would just hit him with anything, and he'd hit me. We'd fight, you know, just like my parents did. It was the same thing, looking back on it, I kind of fell into the same role like my parents, you know, what they would do. They would drink and they would fight, and then I never realized what I was doing." In a similar vein, Louise comments: "I see characteristics in myself that my mother had. Like how far I could push, how far she could push my dad."

Both Theresa and Louise portray active marital violence as involving both their husbands and themselves and as clearly linked to drinking, and they do not explicitly specify serious physical consequences. But younger women describe many variations in the types and levels of domestic violence that they have experienced.

Others describe more serious physical consequences but still position marital violence as situational—related to emotional outbursts while using alcohol, for example. Still others describe more one-sided and entrenched forms of violence, which sometimes involved alcohol but often extended well beyond drinking episodes. The relationship dynamics involved here often appear to involve deeper, more entrenched power politics. These stories parallel some older women's discussions of jealous and controlling husbands but emphasize the emotional dimensions of these experiences.

Heather offers a detailed account of interacting with a violent and controlling husband.

And I used to drink with him, and it seemed like—well, I guess when you have that alcohol, you kind of get brave too? And he was way bigger than me, and I would start arguing with him back, and he would—mostly it would be like [accusations of unfaithfulness], "How come you were with this one?" And he went out on me a lot. Like, I was always the last one to know, some woman had his kid, and then

I would ask him "Is that your kid?" and he would deny it. But [when he accused me] we would really get into it. Well, I'd get the worst end of it, you know, and, boy, I'd have black eyes. . . . Then, when he would sober up, he was just all—he never said he was sorry, you know, after he would see my face. He would act like it didn't happen. And then he would be nice, he was really nice. Like, you know, that alcohol just made him like that.

While the husband's jealous accusations and the links between these, his violence, and alcohol are certainly reminiscent of older women's accounts, Heather offers far more detail about confronting her husband over his infidelity—including details about the scope of her husband's violence, and feelings of fear and worthlessness that it generated within her. She continues:

I used to be really scared of him, and he would kind of threaten me, "Well, you go to your grandpa's or you go to your brother's, I'm going to really beat them up too." So that kind of prevented me from going for help, and at that time they didn't have any help for people like safe houses, now we have battered houses [women's shelters], you know, we never had those. And then there would be times when I would turn him in, and he would go to court, and he would have friends there who would put a wrong date on there, or he would have a friend say, "Well, he was with me," and it would get thrown out. And I would say, "Gee, I can't even find help any place." Sometimes I always wish that I had been a lot stronger and I had moved away from him, or I had left him. How he would put me down. . . . he always made me feel he was the only one ever wanted me.

Heather clearly depicts the fear involved in having kin and institutional supports manipulated out of reach, and the emotional qualities of continuing dependence that resulted (how he "made me feel"). The psychological texture of these forms of intimate partner violence and the feelings of fear and unworthiness that they engendered are echoed by numerous other younger women, who also convey entrenched patterns of control and manipulation in their relationships with boyfriends and husbands.

Some younger women directly link marital violence and instability to their own drinking as adults. As Jackie describes:

One night he was trying to hit me again, and I just fought him and I ran out, and I got caught and thrown in [jail] for being drunk. I was in for [about five days]. So I got out, caught a ride, came home, and looked at my house. I kind of had a lump in my throat 'cause I had all kinds of beer cans, wine bottles laying around; my record player was still going, there were lights on. My door was open, and it was just cold in that house. So I started cleaning it and built a fire in that stove. I went across to my neighbor's and asked if they seen [my husband]. She said "Sit down," and she got some whiskey. She said, "You better sit down and have a drink, because what I'm going to tell you is going to break your heart." I said, "Oh, yeah?" So I drank it down, and she said, "Your husband's with another woman, since the time you been throwed in. . . ." [In the months that followed] I'd stay sober one day, and next day I'm hitch-hiking to town to get drunk.

Others do not describe drinking as a response to men's violence or infidelity, but portray how working to manage the consequences of their husband's behavior became a serious drain on their time and energy. Louise particularly emphasizes her frustration and unhappiness as she tried in various ways to manage her husband's drinking and its consequences:

I used to leave him a lot because of his drinking, but he would always come back and promise me all kinds of things and that he wasn't going to do this and do that, and it would be good again for, like, three, four months. And then it would be the same again. A long time ago I used to call in for him, when we first got together. We fought about [this] a lot, is he wouldn't go to work because of his drinking. It interfered in his work, but then he wouldn't take a day off to take my kids to clinic. He'd say, "I have to work, I can't just be taking time off." So I quit calling in for him. . . . I don't know, I guess I started hating him for choosing alcohol over us, me and my kids. [And] like I'd cook and he'd come home and eat, and other times he wouldn't come, and he'd [call and] say, "I just came down to have a beer." And then I would get mad. I didn't know that was a game. You know, he'd call me up to get me mad. And then later on he said, "Well, you were already mad anyway, so why should I come home?"

Here, Louise documents her frustration with her husband's behavior, but the storyline does not fit that of the failed provider described by so many older women. The husband is consistently employed here, and what frustrates Louise is his willingness to sacrifice for alcohol but not for her or the kids. A Twelve Step–influenced notion of alcohol addiction is clearly central in her portraits of both her husband and herself, especially in her description of her husband's heavy focus on alcohol and on his behavior as a "game" that he initiates to provide himself with excuses for drinking.

The content themes of younger women's discussions of their troubled relationships with men are broadly similar to those of older women, indicating a generally shared understanding that marriage and family are central components of women's social roles. But the forms of their accounts differ substantially. Rhetorics that explicitly attribute relationship troubles to alcohol permeate younger women's accounts. This explanatory emphasis is also apparent in younger women's descriptions of raising children.

Raising Children in Challenging Contexts

Younger women's narratives of becoming parents commonly portray how they reproduced behaviors from their own childhood but, ultimately, came to reflect upon what they were doing. For example, Karen describes her move to awareness in realizing that she was treating her own daughter with the same violence that had caused her so much pain as a child: "I mean, my anger was getting so bad where I'd get mad [at my daughter] and slap her on the arm or kick her butt and say, 'Get in the other room.' You know, and she would cry and it got to the point where I'd hear her crying and I would say, 'Gosh, I'm just—that was just like me [when I was small].'" Many go on to describe how sobriety included reconsidering their behavior and actively seeking alternatives to what they had experienced from their parents (see below).

Echoing older women, younger women also emphasize the special challenges of raising children in family and community contexts of marked substance use and violence. Younger women offer somewhat more detailed examples of encountering family and community members who promote substance use among children. As noted previously, Jeanne describes her frustration over how her siblings would encourage her children to drink and smoke. Rather than always describing such direct causal associations as role-modeling behavior, however, other younger women stress how the conditions of reservation life include multiple threats to the well-being of children that fuel escalating cycles of substance use in each new generation. Rhonda recalls a period in her life in which she divorced her husband, and he threatened to kill her, so she had to call the police and have him thrown in jail. She then took a full-time job to support herself and her children and was having a younger male relative babysit for her kids, when she discovered that the boy had tried to molest one of her children. In taking action to manage one problem, she had created another and experienced extreme stress and frustration as a result: "I really thought I was going to fall apart. I just couldn't take it anymore." Rhonda expresses her central concern as protecting her children from damaging experiences that could lead them into substance abuse.

Many younger women also speak of the frustrations of living in a community in which public institutions to protect well-being do not always function effectively. Many mention the justice system in this regard, noting how known abusers can continue to freely participate in social life on the reservation. As Alice describes: "[A female juvenile relative] was sexually abused, and it was a family member. We've talked to the family, we've talked to the authorities, we've done everything that we're supposed to do. We have family get-togethers and we watch our kids constantly, because this person is still there."[2]

Some women also discuss how marginalization in a racialized social order can impact Northern Cheyenne children. Susan describes trying to comprehend her teenaged son's intense feeling of his own oppression as a Native American in the United States:

> There was so much rage in him, so much hurt, and he tried to explain it, but I couldn't quite grasp what he was saying. There was this white-man kind of game with different minorities, and it's like he already feels doomed or oppressed. I didn't realize that it could bother him that much. It surprised me that he was able to grasp that concept and feel like it was crushing him—what he's struggling against, being from a reservation, being a Native American and being a minority.

With this kind of commentary, younger women describe the continuing vulnerability of their children to a variety of wider social processes and often emphasize how the psychological dimensions of these threats place children at risk for substance abuse.

Rhetorical Tools and Social Experience

For older women, the idiom of forgetting permeates their accounts of witnessing and participating in a decline from the moral world of their earlier childhood in their progression into adulthood. Younger women rely heavily on the Twelve Step idiom of cycles of addiction to portray the reproduction of childhood worlds of disruption and pain in adulthood. What their contrasts highlight is how the conventional local rhetoric of the empty center at Northern Cheyenne, and the ethnopsychological understandings that underwrite this rhetoric, focuses only on learning in childhood as the foundation for identity in adulthood. But this perspective does not acknowledge the force of disruptions experienced by younger women. Younger women's use of elements of Twelve Step discourse may well reflect an effort to construct an alternative vision of Cheyenne personhood. Many younger women emphasize the possibilities for recovery from the cultural disruptions that have impacted Cheyenne family life by linking their personal experiences to accounts of the community's collective history. As Ellen explains: "I started recovering in codependency, and looking back at my family, that's where I realized that all those teaching were already there, my grandparents. It was still sitting there waiting for you. It was like this generation [of my parents] that's stuck." Ellen and many other younger women are aware of theories of historical trauma and its intergenerational consequences through reading recovery materials developed by and for Native Americans, and/or through attending local community workshops based on the Gathering of Native Americans curriculum (see chapter 1). Like Ellen, many found these to be highly resonant with their own experiences, and to affirm their own capacities to critique how the behaviors of some members of older generations on the reservation had impacted family life.

Northern Cheyenne women's descriptions and commentary about family life provide evidence of how subjective experiences on the reservation can be gendered, highlighting how psychological investment in valued caregiving roles for women has shaped how many women think, feel, and respond to experiences of family life. Women's accounts also include critical social commentary about other gender- or age-based social groups, including men, children, and, on occasion, older generations. These critiques demonstrate the complex interweaving of psychological and sociopolitical themes in Northern Cheyenne women's narratives and exemplifies how talk can reflect multiple dimensions of experience as well as multiple goals: to express suffering, to identify its causes, and to potentially legitimate one's own capacities to call for change. The following chapter considers how Northern Cheyenne women's accounts of becoming sober further illuminate the intertwining psychological and sociopolitical stakes involved as women desire and enact changes in their drinking behavior on the reservation, and further emphasizes the differences in perspective and motivation that seem to underwrite the distinctive rhetorical tools that Northern Cheyenne women from different generations use to talk about their life experiences.

6
Narratives of Sobriety
Reconfiguring the Empty Center

Both older and younger women's narratives construct alcohol as a powerful source of disruption in their personal and community worlds and portray sobriety as a difficult but necessary moral reordering of their lives. Yet, in keeping with the rhetorical frameworks discussed in the preceding two chapters, older women describe becoming sober as a return to values that they already knew, often with limited elaboration. In contrast, younger women portray sobriety as an extended process of psychological transformation that involves a detailed process of working through painful emotions and learning about their cultural heritage. Here again, it is clear that older women engage a prevalent and locally conventionalized "rhetoric of the empty center" (O'Nell 1996:55) in describing sobriety as a move toward an idealized past, while younger women draw from a different discursive repertoire that includes terms and concepts from A.A. and related Twelve Step therapies. But younger women's narratives of sobriety also demonstrate how they weave together elements from these different rhetorical resources. Their accounts of sobriety use local rhetorical conventions that construct the past as a moral center for contemporary Cheyenne life but ultimately move to reconfigure them by measuring the distance from the past in terms of a Twelve Step–influenced notion of emotional health.

In these ways, younger women's narratives of sobriety highlight how their use of Twelve Step terms, concepts, and practices is both selective and creative, shaped by their historically contextualized social experiences and subjectivities. These processes are perhaps most evident in their critical appraisals of the Twelve Steps, which enrich and extend the broader local critiques described previously.

Northern Cheyenne women's experiences and stories underscore how there are multiple forms of sobriety on the reservation, each involving different meanings, behaviors, direct social consequences, and broader political implications. This local diversity has clear implications for sobriety

promotion efforts. The politics among these different paths toward sobriety are especially evident in community responses to efforts by some
younger women to integrate Twelve Step approaches with the ongoing
broader local trend toward revitalizing Cheyenne spiritual practices.

Older Women: Sobriety as a Return to Known Values

Older women's narratives of why and how they became sober convey a
general sense of coming back to values and priorities that they knew were
important all along, after a foray into a world that was easy and accessible but had consequences they did not like. In describing how they came
to desire a sober life, some cite specific experiences with legal problems,
such as arrests for alcohol-related charges (e.g., public intoxication, DUI).
Others position health concerns as a major motivation. Rosemary links
her own experiences with the unpleasant aftereffects of drinking to her
observations of other women in the community who died of cirrhosis,
and how she came to conclude that she was risking a similar fate: "[After
drinking] next day I would have a hangover. I couldn't handle it. If I had
kept going, I would be gone now—from cirrhosis. Like [names a peer and
friend]—she really went fast, from drinking, after her husband left her for
another girl. Her mother died from liver problems too, from drinking."

Yet older women most commonly reference family responsibilities
as motivations for sobriety. Mary expresses how she and her husband
would sometimes drink in front of their children, and how her husband recurrently became violent in front of them. Invoking a prominent
local developmental model of teaching and learning, she emphasizes her
concern about what such spectacles were teaching her children: "I was
taught that drinking families were no good. I think that's one of the reasons I didn't drink [heavily]—that was in my mind all the time. I never
craved it; I just quit. I didn't want my kids to see me drinking."

In a similarly structured account, Laura describes how she was motivated to quit drinking by a combination of factors, but especially by the
desire to set a good example for her daughter.

> I got tired of bumming. I wanted a job and I wanted to keep it. I
> got one, but I still drank sometimes too. My daughter went away to
> school, really worked hard. She would call home. Then one time she
> said, "I can never get a hold of you, you're out drunk. I'll just come
> home and join you—be a drunk too." I cried and said, "No, don't do

that!" I said, "I'll quit," and I did. Some say they crave it—if they see beer, or someone drinking. It doesn't bother me. I never craved for a smoke either. I don't know how that feels.

Here, Laura emphasizes how her choice to be sober first involved pulling back from nonreciprocal modes of exchange like "bumming," and focusing instead on holding down a job. Under pressure from her daughter, she then fully confronted her desire to be a role model for a productive and hardworking way of living.

Like Mary, Laura portrays sobriety as a process of remembering and returning to values that she already knew. Also like Mary, she explicitly states that she did not "crave" alcohol when she quit. Mary, Laura, and other older women emphasize that, for them, the most painful consequence of quitting drinking was not the loss of a relationship with alcohol, but the loss of their former drinking friends.

Older Women and Sobriety: Facing the Social Consequences

Older women recurrently stress the importance of the courage and determination required to resist pressure from their former drinking friends. In an account that reflects a prominent local ethnopsychological understanding that a person is open to influence by others (Straus 1977), Martha describes personal resolve and a conscious effort to avoid her former companions as essential components of her sobriety: "I made up my mind, and I just quit on my own. I stayed away [from my former drinking friends]." Laura offers more detail about how her choice to quit drinking generated considerable social pressure.

People started calling me down. "Angel, perfect woman, she doesn't want to drink with us." I would say, "No one offers me beer or money when I have a hangover, but I hustle for all of you. You have no one to hustle for you now." I lost all my friends. I would still talk to good friends, encourage them to quit—no more hangovers. But they call me down, talk about me behind my back. So I am alone. I say, "Hi, how are you," but it's not like before.

Here, Laura emphasizes how her drinking friends accused her of violating local ethics of egalitarianism, and how she responded by pointing out how their own behavior violates local ethics of reciprocity.

The result has been hurtful talk ("calling me down"), even as Laura has tried to encourage a shift to sobriety or to continue social pleasantries with her former drinking buddies.

Josephine seems to have spent considerable time and energy considering the nature and dynamics of social exclusion in sobriety. She tells a story about how at one point after she stopped drinking, she found herself wanting to seek out her former drinking friends:

> You're an outsider once you quit. You don't belong anymore. So I'd go over there, and we'd sit in there and, you know, we'd talk like, "Gee, remember that time we ran off the road?" or "Remember that time we beat this girl up?" and we'd laugh and she'd be sitting there drinking, and she'd say, "Come on, Josie, drink," you know. And there are times when I'm ready to reach out. Because it was going so good, you know, the stories—the things that we experienced together. Sometimes they start getting mean, you know. "Gee, Josie thinks she's somebody just because she quit." Where they just say, "Well, why don't you just leave, you know, you don't belong here anymore," or "We don't need you here any more—you're no fun," you know. And then I just walked out. I guess she said, "All that time she's thinking 'Oh, these poor ladies, I'm glad I'm not, you know, I'm not in your shoes anymore.'"

Again, her friends accuse her of violating an ethic of egalitarianism in seeing herself as "perfect" or "thinking you're somebody" for quitting. The experience of isolation associated with sobriety is embodied as they ask her to leave.

Sobriety as Courage

Older women generally describe how they came to see how their drinking lives lacked the esteemed values that shaped the worlds of their early childhoods, such as courage and resilience in the face of difficulty. As Ruth describes, from this perspective frustration and self-pity figure prominently in motives for continued drinking: "The ones I have seen—they drink when there's a death in the family. When they get drunk, they bring it up—loss of that relative. They have a drinking problem now. They don't want to help themselves, even though they have their own families. The ones that are unemployed get discouraged when they don't get hired, start drinking. When they run into difficulty, they drink."

In discussing how transformations in priorities helped them to avoid continued drinking, many older women describe with emotion how their family responsibilities motivated them to stop drinking, and like Ruth many associated drinking with emotional states of grief or discouragement in response to life's difficulties. Their narratives cast sobriety as a process centered on knowledge they already had, coupled with the courage to act despite suffering serious social consequences. Prominent local rhetorics that contrast past with present are evident in how many older women invest moral value in living closer to a more coherent past. Notably, older women's accounts do not include highly detailed discussion of how they stopped drinking, reference to novel ways of understanding themselves or their world that accompanied this change, or other themes prominent within Twelve Step approaches.

Yet an awareness of Twelve Step understandings of sobriety is visible in older women's narratives. Several remark that they do not know what it feels like to "crave" alcohol. Laura states a clear consciousness ("Some say they crave it") of alternative perspectives in the community that are centered on such notions of addiction. While these perspectives are most visibly developed in the narratives of younger women, several older women did describe learning about Twelve Step concepts and practices through their employment experiences or through attending treatment centers as family members to support younger relatives seeking help there.

Older Women and Twelve Step Recovery

Martha describes how new knowledge gained from a job as an alcohol counselor, entering a new social world as she remarried, and legal consequences from drinking all converged in her decision to quit drinking: "I quit on my own. I made up my mind to do it. I started working as a counselor, got training. Then I met my husband, who is sober and who knew about alcoholism. I came to see then why my other marriages didn't work out. There was quite a bit of abuse. At the time I did not see it as related to alcohol. I sometimes fell off the wagon after that, but then I got a DUI, and I just quit." Martha talks about what she learned about alcoholism here but begins and ends her discussion by emphasizing that she quit on her own—as she notes, through a combination of making up her mind and being tired of the negative consequences of drinking.

Similarly, Esther describes an encounter with Twelve Step concepts and practices that was helpful, but brief: "My daughter went to treatment, and I went with her. She cried and cried. The counselors kept us over one week, because it was so hard to break me down, for me to admit that I had a problem. I finally broke down and cried, and just let all my feelings out. It did wonders—has kept me going ever since. I find that in hard times, I go to prayer meetings, or somewhere where I can feel closer to God." She portrays her use of a formal treatment program as a one-time event and explains how she does not continue to use such resources but relies on others instead.

Yet most older women did not specifically mention Twelve Step concepts or practices. As a founding member of the first Northern Cheyenne women's Alcoholics Anonymous group, Josephine was the major exception. Instead, the most well-developed ideas about addiction, the psychological effects of violence, and unhealthy attachments to people necessitating a long-term process of recovery are visible in younger women's narratives. Younger women often portray sobriety as a major process, involving learning about addiction and the nature and management of their own emotional lives—and also about their local cultural heritage as Northern Cheyennes.

Younger Women: Sobriety as Personal Growth

Younger women depict sobriety as fundamentally an educational process, a process of unlearning the destructive ways of thinking, feeling, and behaving that they had adopted, and replacing them with more positive, constructive patterns through a conscious and reflexive process of self-education. This process of learning new skills was so extensive that in explaining it, younger women frequently draw analogies to a process of maturing. Pauline says: "It's like growing up—growing up all over again. That's how I look at it—learning to do this, and learning to do that. Because no one ever taught me them skills, when I was small." Sharla echoes: "I think I've grown up a lot, you know? Let things go—they are not mine any more, all the times I've been abused or hurt or whatever. Now I'm an adult, I'm in the next stage of my life. Things can hurt me, but they don't have to overwhelm me."

This notion of extensive psychological transformation is especially central within ACOA and codependency therapies' constructions of recovery. Several younger women explicitly identify how they learned these Twelve Step terms and concepts though experiences at Recovery Center and/or in treatment. Yet younger women are also highly critical of some dimensions of the Twelve Step approaches and use them selectively.

Younger Women: Motives for Recovery

Younger women's discussions of what provoked this process were often broadly similar to older women's: they were sick of the consequences of alcohol in their lives and came to recognize how drinking was interfering with desired goals. Some mention health issues, like Stephanie, who emphasizes how for her sobriety came in phases. First, tired of the consequences and responsive to family concern, she drastically reduced the frequency with which she drank. Later, she was inspired to quit for a much longer time period by a brush with a serious illness.

> My sister would say, "You should stop drinking and come back home, 'cause you're really getting Mom worried." And I was telling her, I said, "Well, I'm not ready yet." And then that one whole week we started drinking just nothing but tequila, and, man, that was just like every day, tequila, tequila, tequila bottles all over . . . lemon peels, salt shakers all over. The whole house was just a party house and stuff, and people I didn't even know. Boy, I was hung over for what felt like three days or something. And after I finally got over that hangover, then that's when I called home, and I told them that I want to come back now. It just started getting old, like, what's the use, you know? [Drank on and off after that point, but then suffered a serious illness.] Then I kind of saw life differently. Time to get serious here—I'm going to stop playing around, get serious and figure out what I want to do and what it is I'm supposed to be doing.

A number of younger women also mention how alcohol impacted their ability to pursue other valued goals, such as education. As Pauline describes:

> I woke up one morning, I was so hung over. . . . Then I knew I had ran out of excuses—I could feel it in my body. I had to do something. That was where I was, when I hit bottom. I had enrolled in college, and my grades were going down, and I started realizing that my using and college life just wasn't working for me. So, I decided to go to treatment.

And for some reason I really felt sincere, you know, like this was really time for me to find a different life.

Both Pauline and Stephanie mention the significance of cultivating a new sense of purpose in their lives as an important support for sobriety—a sense that there was something better for them to be doing with their time and energy than drinking, and that they needed to figure out exactly what that was.

While these notions of exploration are absent from older women's narratives, younger women with children did similarly emphasize caregiving responsibilities as a motive for sobriety. As Jenny describes:

I realized that I was taking my children through a lot of hardship, undue misery. Many times I'd get off a drunk and look in the 'fridge, and there'd be nothing there for us to eat. I had an aunt that would bring me food and feed my children, and I began to realize that that wasn't right either, that I had been using up all my paycheck to drink. After my [last months] of drinking I really desperately was looking for a change in my life. I just got down on my knees and prayed all night, and I just cried and asked the Creator. . . . I had a lot of confusion about who the Creator was, God or Ma?heo?o. [But] I asked for a better life, a good life. I wanted to be able to take care of my children in a good way, raise them good.

Yet, instead of older women's portrayal of a relatively clean and clear break from a negative life, with the major price being social isolation, Jenny's story emphasizes her feelings of confusion. Notably here, she references the same spiritual confusion that she previously attributed to her grandfather in her account of young adulthood.

Jenny also goes on to describe how, while Twelve Step approaches were not entirely sufficient to support her sobriety, she did find significant help from them. She went to treatments for both drinking and codependency, as did most of the younger women I interviewed. While others did not, they gained information about various Twelve Step therapies from reading Twelve Step literature and talking with relatives and friends who attended meetings. While their familiarity with the terminology, concepts, and practices varies, the overwhelming majority of younger women voice common features and goals of Twelve Step recovery, such as developing new skills for dealing with painful emotions and difficult life situations and, centrally, for talking about feelings.

Sobriety as Psychological Transformation

Many younger women describe how Twelve Step frameworks and activities have provided them with a useful new vocabulary and, alongside it, a new appreciation of the importance of talk in the therapeutic resolution of painful emotions that would have previously provoked a bout of drinking or cycles of unfulfilling attachments to abusive and/ or addicted people.

Some describe how the Twelve Steps helped them to identify what they had always felt but never clearly understood before. Recall Louise's comments: "Going to treatment was one of the best things I ever done for myself, because I learned a lot that I never knew before. I grieved for my grandmother for years, and I didn't even know it. . . . I felt that abandonment and—well, you see I didn't know all these words 'til I went to treatment." Similarly, Theresa says, "I never even knew about the inner child until I went over there [to Recovery Center]. Working on myself and how to enjoy myself more and do things for myself instead of, you know—I was doing things for everybody [else]." Echoing classic formulations of consciousness raising, Susan describes learning to name an inchoate problem:

> After you learn about alcoholism, there's just so many dysfunctional behaviors that go along with it that nobody can have a healthy marriage or a healthy relationship with their husband or with their kids, with their family, with loved ones, with anybody. . . . it just destroys you mentally, emotionally, physically, spiritually. And after learning about that I just always kind of knew, "Hey, this is not right—what's happening in my life and my family." I knew it wasn't right. I just didn't have the knowledge . . . or I couldn't identify it with words, but after I started learning, then I could look back [and see that] it came from alcoholism.

In contrast to older women who portrayed how they already knew that something was wrong in their drinking lives, Susan portrays not having a clear frame of reference from childhood to make such determinations. Nonetheless, she "felt" it was wrong and positions a Twelve Step definition of alcoholism as an authoritative standard of what constitutes emotional well-being. By providing her with the power to identify and talk about problems, this resource helped her to work toward enacting such standards in her life.

Jenny uses a metaphor of movement to describe this process of burgeoning awareness and action, noting that new skills of self-reflection freed her to go with the flow of life in healthier and more constructive ways:

> Recovery to me means taking a look at issues that are weighing you down or that are keeping you stuck—to take a look at them and deal with them. Because a lot of these issues, they hold us down and they keep us from going to what we can be. I didn't know, but I had a lot of anger and rage from my childhood, living in an alcoholic home. In therapy I was able to take them out, take a look at them, deal with them, you know. . . . But I had a lot of fear of people that hurt me when I was little. It just kind of gave me a sense of freedom, that I could finally let go of the past and look forward to the future. It's helped me to open up my mind and expand.

She again emphasizes the extensive learning process involved here, as well as the centrality of feelings of anger and fear in her previous life. A key theme in Jenny's narrative of learning to manage these feelings involves coming to terms with her painful experiences with her parents. She notes how the Twelve Step conceptualization of addiction as a disease enabled her to work through these feelings and come to a sense of forgiveness: "I was able to learn about the addiction of alcohol and drugs, and the power. Learning about the disease itself really helped me to see why my life had been the way it was. I was able to see how my mom and dad were affected by it, so I was able to forgive them and move on, just knowing that they suffered too from the disease, and it hindered them from giving us children a good life."

Indeed, most younger women similarly emphasized the importance of talk as part of learning to consciously feel and "work through" painful emotions. As Pauline remarks: "Coming into recovery was something I learned how to do. Because I never learned to get in touch with my feelings before, because I was never taught, and I was brought up in a dysfunctional family, you know—don't talk, don't trust, don't feel, those were the three rules that I was brought up with. After I got into recovery, I started learning how to get in touch with my emotions and how to work through them." Here, "don't talk, don't trust, don't feel" explicitly references Adult Children of Alcoholics author Claudia Black's (2001) formulation of the unspoken but powerful rules of an alcoholic family.

Younger women stress how talking about feelings and problems has offered ways of resolving difficulties in their lives, rather than unsuccessfully trying to ignore or avoid them through drinking. As Jeanne explains: "The problems that you encounter, especially if you're using, they seem like they're big problems, real big, and you go drink—you still have that problem. At least when you're sober as each day goes by, it's nothing. You think back, it's just a little problem, little petty thing. But when you're drinking or using drugs, feeling like you got no help—you think it's just big. But there's always help. Talking it out, it helps." Younger women especially emphasize the importance of talk for healing from intensely painful experiences that generated powerful negative emotions such as hatred and shame. Sexual abuse serves as a prominent example here. Amanda says: "The first thing you need to do is tell who it was, because you're so ashamed and that's power over you. I was able to confront the man who molested me and tell him what kind of effect he'd had on my life. He cried and told me that he had been abused himself. That didn't excuse what he did, but confronting him helped me to move on, out of that pain."

In addition to confronting an abuser, younger women portray talk and positive social interactions with others in recovery as important in supporting their sobriety. Kim describes how such experiences improved the "self-esteem" that she needed to overcome feelings of shame:

I was embarrassed about the way I was living, and I didn't know how to deal with it. Having other people to talk to was really helpful. They give you feedback—not like advice so much as reassurance. Going to meetings and having that support really made me feel good and boosted my self-esteem. I think that talking about my problems and realizing that they weren't so terrible helped me with my self-esteem. I could feel good about myself.

Many younger women also describe how they took their newfound communication skills and applied them to their lives at home and work, improving the quality of their relationships and their own sense of well-being. As Andrea reports: "When me and my husband have problems, before it gets super-angry, I tell him 'Just go.' We'll talk when we calm down instead of screaming at each other at the top of our lungs. I don't want [my children] to see that. [My husband] goes outside and works on his truck or on another car, or he'll go for a walk. When we cool off, we try to talk about it." Pauline describes how practicing these skills could be challenging but was ultimately rewarding, because it reduced conflict in her relationships and generally enhanced her feelings of well-being.

> I have changed from my old behavior of dealing with problems, and found new ways, healthier ways, of dealing with problems. And it's better that way—I don't have to carry grudges and resent this one or that one, like I did before. Now I can work through my problems and let them go. There's still times I'll say something that wasn't nice of me to say. I'll go back and apologize. And let it go, you know, instead of staying mad at this person. . . . when I do confront an issue, I feel a lot better. I guess it's that feeling of feeling better that gives me the urge to do it, to keep doing it.

These discussions of talk and emotion in younger women's narratives are similar to stories of Twelve Step recovery in many nonindigenous contexts. But as younger women talk about sobriety, it is also clear that many relate the scope and nature of their emotional difficulties to the localized context of their lives as Native American women living on a reservation.

Local Particulars: Personal Experience and Collective History

Some women describe how implementing a conventional Twelve Step recovery process has been difficult for them, given the conflicts that it can produce with locally valued kinship responsibilities. Jeanne relates incidences of conflict with her siblings and other family members on these grounds, as she came into sobriety.

> My nephews, two of my nephews, they'd come up to the house, my grandpa would bring them, and he would say, "She's drinking again. I don't think they ate," you know. Oh, I'd just get really mad and kind of get mad at my grandfather, too, and say, "Don't be taking them. She has to take care of them. We're just, you know, like, enabling her to keep on, 'cause she knows they've got a place to go." So I would think like that, but then on the other hand, they were my nephews,

you know, and I wanted to take care of them too. So I would really get mad at her, and then she would get mad and wouldn't talk to me for a while, wouldn't come around.

Younger women also identify the ways in which kinship intersects with frequent violence and alcohol on the reservation to produce uniquely powerful feelings of grief, and how deaths of family and community members derive further significance from a locally distinctive sense of history. As Julia and Ellen variously comment,

> On the outside, people die when they are older, so their relatives are prepared for it and can grieve. With the violence and alcohol ongoing here, you can never finish grieving before the next accident or death. And any death affects the whole tribe, not just the family, because we are such a small community. (Julia)

> Here, everybody grieves for the elders [when] they die, because they know how much they're taking with them; they're going to miss them because they're so much a part of your life to the end. (Ellen)

For Julia and Ellen, the sheer level of community violence, the kinship system, and the unique local value placed on the cultural knowledge of older generations emerge as particular sources of loss for Northern Cheyenne community members.

Some younger women also discuss how their hopes that their own recovery would positively impact their families have faced special challenges on the reservation. Susan and Pauline acknowledge the normative nature of substance use and related problems in the community but articulate hope that their sobriety could bring change:

> It's a part of life for a lot of people. But with each of our generations, we're addressing it more and more and learning about it and taking positive steps to, you know, where it might not exist in my children's lives. We're teaching our children to be more open to recovery, to reach out for help. (Susan)

> I'm glad today that I can talk to my kids about this stuff that happened, you know, the domestic abuse, the sexual abuse. Everything that was a secret at that time. I can talk about it now, openly, with

my kids, and tell them this is where we're going to break this cycle. (Pauline)

Yet many younger women convey a profound awareness of the difficulties posed by the fact that their children are influenced by many factors beyond one or both of their parents' recovery. Many emphasize how the locally normative nature of drinking and drug use influences their children, and the stresses of living in conditions that pose multiple threats to well-being. Many emphasize their frustration at how this context produces problems among their children and grandchildren in spite of their own sobriety. Theresa says:

> When I stopped drinking, I thought, "Well, like a cycle, it's got to stop someplace." And I said, "I want it to stop here, for my family." But it didn't, even now my son is doing it. And it's already into my grandchildren. Sometimes I go get my grandchildren, 'cause I don't want to see them in that kind of [drinking] environment. And my one grandson is a real angry little boy, 'cause his parents drink and they don't . . . he's already trying to be on his own, he won't even listen to them.

To begin to address some of these special local issues, some younger women make use of elements of the historical/multigenerational trauma models popularized by key mental health researchers and national organizations devoted to Native American sobriety (e.g., Coyhis and White 2002; Duran and Duran 1995). Alice describes how she came to forgive her parents through historically situating their experiences in the context of forced assimilation:

> They were raised in boarding schools; they didn't know how to be parents. They had never had the parenting to learn how to be traditional, or the culture, because they were with nuns and priests who were trying to change them, not to be Indian, and I guess that's the shame that they carried on to me. I used to hate my mom and dad and wonder why is our life so screwed up, how come they couldn't be better parents to me, and then it took becoming a parent myself to finally realize that they never had a chance to be parents. So I did a lot of forgiving of them then, because they couldn't give what they didn't have.

Becky discusses this process of forgiveness most extensively, in relation to her family experiences but also in relation to coming to terms with Christianity, in a process that she wryly terms becoming a "recovering Catholic." She first offers a detailed account of an important conversation with her father:

> I asked my dad one day, "How come you sent us to Catholic school, they were really mean to us over there." He just sat there and listened to me, and he was real quiet, and then he said, "Well, we were still coming out of the Depression when you were born. . . . do you think we wanted to do that? Nobody wanted to do that, but then nobody could feed all those kids." He also told me how at that point in his life, his priority was drinking, rather than his family . . . and he said, "I feel really bad about it now, but there's no way I can go back and change what I did." And so conversations like that from him really helped me to understand why I was there.

Becky goes on to describe how she actually attended an informal discussion group at the Catholic mission where she had gone to school as a child, in which she was able to voice her experiences to former teachers and to learn about their own perspectives.

> And those people at the school, they were doing what they thought was right at the time. . . . their job was to take the Indian out of you, and they did that. And I was a victim of that, and I lived in that era. So when I go back and I think about what their job was, and I guess that's how I forgave. . . . And I think that they were ordered to do that, and a lot of times I don't think that they did it out of their own vindictiveness. Some might have, but I don't think all of them were that way. [Because] they changed. By the time I was in seventh and eighth grade, things had changed there—they became less rigid, and less harsh in their discipline. [As an adult] I talked to some nuns who were recovering Catholics themselves. . . . I got the inside story of Vatican I and how it changed over to Vatican II and how more liberal they became. And they were in those stages themselves, and, you know, they had to be real disciplined themselves. And they got beat by people that were in authority in their institutions. And, you know, and some of them admitted that they were running away from home because of their own sexual abuse.

Here, Becky contextualizes the behavior of the nuns and other boarding school staff as the product of a historical process, in which they as well as she were enmeshed. Framing the nuns' behavior as learned in response to both institutional and personal violence helps to make it intelligible in new ways that, for Becky, blunt its ability to continue generating fear, anger, and other painful emotions.

Younger women also highlight the limits of the Twelve Step emphasis on a spiritual foundation for sobriety, noting that it was helpful but not culturally specific in the ways that they needed and wanted. Instead, many have looked to Cheyenne ritual practices such as sweat lodges, fasting, and peyote meetings as key resources in supporting their sobriety (see also Baird-Olsen and Ward 2000; Bezdek and Spicer 2006; Medicine 2007). Karen describes her sense that Twelve Step methods and practices alone left her feeling in need of something more: "When I got out of treatment, I made a commitment to fast. That was our traditional way, to go to a tipi and fast. It was like I was searching, I was searching for something. When I went to treatment, it was like you have a sore and you pour salt on it." Jenny's encounters with Alcoholics Anonymous coincided with her entry into the Native American Church (NAC, or peyote church). She notes that while she stopped going to A.A. after a time, she continued to attend NAC meetings:

A friend in A.A. kept inviting me to go to meetings with her. Then she let me use one of her books, and I just really identified with it and I read it and began to attend more A.A. meetings. And around that time I had a cousin that kept wanting to take me to Native American Church, and she wouldn't give up on me, and she'd always invite me through the years, but I would never go. I would always have some excuse, 'cause I felt like I didn't belong there. I didn't feel worthy of going. [But] she was really persistent, and she sat by me, and she helped me all night. I just felt a lot of love there, a real positive atmosphere. I seen a lot of real caring people there, and I thought, this is something that I've been searching for all my life. That need to belong—like, hey, I'm an Indian, and I have every right to be an Indian, I have every right to be here, and this is our home, and I really liked that feeling. . . . To this day, I still attend NAC meetings. It's kind of like my anchor, anchor to life here.

Here, Jenny emphasizes that becoming sober involved confronting confusion about who she was and about the legitimacy of her identity as a Native person, and associated feelings of shame. Themes of feeling renewed pride in her cultural heritage, feeling motivated to learn more, and coming to feel "worthy" of being Cheyenne recur throughout her narrative.

Some younger women portray local spiritual practices as things that they had known about earlier in their lives but were unable to fully appreciate while they were drinking. For example, Jeanne describes how her grandfather would try to help her and involve her in peyote meetings as a young adult, and how she would not listen, instead getting caught up in her own life and/or in feeling suspicious of unfamiliar social contexts:

> My grandfather, he used to go to peyote meetings a lot, and he'd tell me to come over and eat. And like he would tell me, "Come back and eat." You know, and I'd think I don't want to go back and eat, they will just say I just came over to eat, you know. And now I realize that it's not like that, they don't think like that, the ones that go to these meetings. And I thought back to what I missed out on, and how I could have hurt my grandfather's feelings, you know. He would come home and say, "They prayed for you," you know, and I would think "So what." You know, it didn't dawn on me, I couldn't really grasp the meaning of what he was saying, and why he would go. And now, now I know, going to the meetings, what I really missed out on.

Yet many younger women emphasize that they had virtually no prior experience with these dimensions of local cultural heritage. Jenny recurrently stresses how she needed to learn more about her Cheyenne heritage and explicitly describes how this learning process and her use of the Twelve Steps were profoundly intertwined.

> The Twelve Steps of A.A. really connects with the Cheyenne way of life. But I more or less took the Cheyenne way, the sweats and peyote meetings and Sun Dances. That's where I get a lot of my strength and guidance and just listening to people talk about the way it used to be a long time ago. The respect that was there, the generosity, and I always try to live by those principles as close as I can, but I'm only human and I can't always fulfill . . . I can never fulfill the way our ancestors used to live, but I always try to live along those lines.

Jenny specifically positions the Twelve Steps as overlapping with "the Cheyenne way" (see also Gone 2008) but emphasizes and privileges the latter as the orienting framework for her life of sobriety.

In these ways, while younger women clearly portray Twelve Step concepts and practices as an important resource in their sobriety, many also describe how their pursuit of sobriety in the context of reservation life raises issues that conventional Twelve Step approaches do not adequately address. The selectivity that they exercise in their use of the Twelve Steps is perhaps clearest in their explicit critiques of some of its key terms and practices.

Selectively Engaging the Twelve Steps

Younger women who describe some elements of the Twelve Steps as very helpful in their sobriety are often openly critical of others. Some of these criticisms echo those that circulate throughout the reservation as a whole. Some younger women respond to the label of "alcoholic" with skepticism, for example, noting that although they were helped by the Twelve Steps, they never believed that they were actually alcoholics. As Evelyn comments, "I don't think I was dependent on alcohol. I didn't need it for my life to work, or run. I was young, and I had problems that I didn't know how to deal with, so I drank to get away from them."

Yet some also raise new issues. Evelyn expresses distaste, for example, for what she sees as individualistic tendencies amongst some Twelve Step adherents:

> Some people in recovery get on a real self-centered kick. Like a woman I know well who has been sober for five years. She goes to meetings and workshops, but she doesn't deal with her kids' complaints or problems. She doesn't give them nurturing and guidance; she is just focused on herself. In treatment they stress that "you're #1"—which is true, but if you have kids you can't be brainwashed that way. You have to think about them. You can be #1, and love yourself, and still realize that you need to love your kids.

As throughout women's narratives, caregiving responsibilities figure here as the ultimate arbiter of appropriate and desirable behavior, especially for women with children.

Still others describe how their understandings of sobriety did not include complete abstinence, as Twelve Step approaches presume, but rather cutting down on the quantity or changing the form of their alcoholic beverages. A few also report plans to limit abstinence to a period in their lives in which other responsibilities are more pressing (e.g., child rearing). In these ways, younger women subvert or ignore central assumptions of conventional Twelve Step approaches, rather than engaging them wholesale.

Generational Contrasts: Rhetoric and Experience

Key differences between older and younger women's accounts of sobriety appear in their discussions of the social consequences of no longer drinking. While older women heavily emphasize the isolation that resulted from their sobriety, younger women describe a broader range of consequences. Some do discuss isolation, as Hannah describes: "You know, ever since I've been sober my life has been pretty boring. But that's OK—it's a peaceful boring. . . . I had a lot of friends when I was drinking. Now I feel lonely. I just go home; nobody comes to visit any more. When I was drinking, someone was always around—never a dull moment!" Yet many offer more detailed discussions of how they reworked key relationships in their lives and/or how their recovery activities helped to generate new social networks.

Some younger women stress that changing relationships was necessary in their sobriety—not just avoiding drinking friends, as older women emphasized, but altering other social relationships, especially with parents, children, and husbands who were drinking and/or leading their lives in unhealthy ways. Becky describes taking the dramatic action of refusing to help her parents while they were drinking, exasperated by their extending this behavior into the home that she was trying to create for her own children.

> There was a point in my life where it was 40 below zero and they called me from the bar, I wouldn't go after them. And finally my mother said, "We're freezing to death up here—we're freezing!" You know, and it was like four o'clock in the morning, so I finally went after them. And after they sobered up—a couple of weeks went by, and I told my mother and dad, I said, "Don't you ever come to my house and drink." I said, "I lived with that all my life, you're not gonna

drink in front of my kids. . . . I refuse to put my kids through the same thing you put me through."

Others report facing tough decisions in their marriages. It is something of a local stereotype, in fact, that a marriage will end if the wife sobers up and the husband does not. Susan references this topic diplomatically, describing her own decision to divorce, but noting how women that she knows actually make a variety of choices in such situations.

> No choice is wrong. I don't think I condemn anybody else's choices if they stay in a relationship like that. You just have to work extra hard, you know? But I let my relationship go because of that. I left their father because I just outgrew—he refused to grow with me. I knew that I wanted to grow further into my recovery, and it just seemed like [he] was not really wanting to learn, but staying sober because I thought it was the right thing to do. He was doing it for me and not for himself. So I made a choice to leave him and take care of myself and my kids. And they know that their father drinks, but they've accepted that he chose that kind of life and their mom chose a different kind of life. But I always encourage [them] not to judge their father. We still get along really good with their father. But I finally realized then that I was beating my head against the wall. I have no control—I have no power over him. So that's when I finally decided to work on myself. . . . hopefully, maybe one of these days I'll meet someone and have a healthy relationship.

A number of women born in the 1960s and later that I interviewed were single due to divorce or because they had never married. Like Susan, many describe a basic contradiction between their conceptualization of a "healthy" relationship and their experiences and available men on the reservation (meaning men not currently involved with other women or considered relatives in Cheyenne modes of reckoning kinship). While older women also criticize men and describe experiences with divorce, they do not commonly articulate these problems in terms of "health." These differences also reflect younger women's far greater investment in articulating a specific vision of emotional well-being.

Some younger women describe how their educational pursuits and attendance at workshops, sweat lodges, and peyote meetings helped them to develop new networks of friends who do not drink. Stephanie and Jenny both use the metaphor of "family" to describe these new connections. As Stephanie reflects: "I've found a different circle of friends. What really helped is the sweats. I like the prayer part in my life—to understand or to know about the sweat lodge or the process of it. And then we get people in there in the sweat lodge, good friends, and they come here and they're a new family, a new prayer family, and it's just really nice. It's a good atmosphere." Many older women, in contrast, simply did not see entering into new ritual activities without having been raised to do so as an option.

In another reflection of the local cultural contextualization of sobriety at Northern Cheyenne, younger women do not only make selective and creative use of the Twelve Steps, but actively weave Twelve Step discourse together with elements of local rhetorical conventions. As with older women, for example, the quotes from Jenny above clearly indicate that she invests her Cheyenne heritage with positive moral value. Her clear privileging of "the way it used to be" and "the Cheyenne way," and her statement that she can only approximate but never fulfill the ways of her ancestors, indicates that she is also employing a rhetoric of the empty center as a discursive tool. Yet her use of this rhetoric is distinct from most older women's in at least three ways.

First, Jenny's descriptions of her sobriety consistently emphasize learning to better manage her emotions in ways consonant with Twelve Step approaches. For example, Jenny speaks of how her spiritual practices helped her to develop patience.

Indian way of prayer takes a lot of patience, 'cause the settings themselves, they teach you to be patient and, like, in the sweat lodge you have to tolerate the hot heat. And then in Sun Dance, going to fast in there, you just sit in there and pray and meditate, and you get hungry, you get restless, but you're in there for a purpose, and your mind has to stay on your purpose, why you went in. Sometimes you get restless and you want it to hurry up and end. But that teaches you patience, and the Native American Church, you know, they're all night long, and sometimes you want it to hurry up and get done, but you have to sit through and be patient. I used to get mad really easy, you know, really get impatient and frustrated. But I've seen a lot and I feel like I've really grown in that area, learning to kind of wait a little bit.

Valuing patience fits well not only with the philosophies of the Native American Church but also with broader local cultural values at Northern Cheyenne, as evidenced in the numerous stories that privilege the reduction of social conflict. Yet Jenny also seems to engage Twelve Step approaches in specifying anger and frustration here. These emotions are centrally problematized in conventional Twelve Step approaches, and Jenny previously described learning to manage them through therapy.

A second difference emerges in Jenny's discussion of needing to over-come feelings of confusion and shame to learn about and participate in her Cheyenne heritage. Rather than referencing a coherent moral world in her early life, Jenny portrays a highly disrupted world and especially identifies psychological and cultural consequences of colonization that are overlooked by how local rhetorical conventions devalue community members with incomplete knowledge of whatever a given speaker defines as tradition. Jenny's own experiences of pain, and of the insufficiencies of prominent local rhetorics for making sense of it, seem evident in her interest in and use of conceptual frameworks of historical trauma.

Older and younger women also differ in their constructions of Cheyenne spiritual practices. Jenny justifies her own increasing partici-pation in these practices, a striking contrast to assertions by some older women that these should be avoided by all but a few ritual specialists. The content of what constitutes tradition varies by generation. Older women emphasize the importance of kinship ties, language, conflict-reducing comportment through calm and respectful talk, and proper ritual pro-tocol. Younger women emphasize active involvement in ritual practices, and conflict reduction through the styles of emotional expression advo-cated by the Twelve Steps.

Reconfiguring the Empty Center:
A Plurality of Local Moral Worlds

By attributing moral authority to both local rhetorical conventions and a Twelve Step–influenced conceptualization of psychological well-being in their narratives, younger women have reconfigured the former by recasting the distance between past and present in emotional terms. This reconfiguration disrupts the usual consequences of this rhetoric in local social life on the reservation, such as naturalizing connections between older age and increased cultural legitimacy (see also O'Nell 1996:65).

Younger women's active interest in ritual practices further challenges local conventions of gender- and generationally based access to these cultural resources, reinterpreting legitimate use of them in terms of emotional maturity and health. By portraying Cheyenne identity as achievable through personal growth, this reconfiguration moves to subvert the totalizing and essentializing ascription of Cheyenne personhood that usually accompanies the use of this rhetoric on the reservation.

The politics associated with younger women's formulations of the links between personhood, identity, and health at Northern Cheyenne can be intense. For example, some younger women explicitly challenge the legitimacy of claims by "traditional" community members by identifying unresolved emotional dimensions of addiction among them, including anger, bitterness, vengefulness, and destructive criticism. As Pauline comments: "It seems like to me, there's traditional people in the community here who are negative, who still put other people down. But for me, I learned that you try not to be negative, you try to see the positive side of a person. That's what I learned in my recovery." Jackie articulates similar themes:

> People can say anything to my uncle, and he won't get mad. He'll just say "Ha-ho [expression for "thank you" across northern Plains tribes], thank you for saying that to me. I'm glad that's how you feel about me." That's a man I admire; that's a traditional way. But most people, it seems like they just get mad right back. And some people, it's like they do it [participate in spiritual practices] to show off. And I don't like people like that, people that use it like that. And there's a lot of other things that goes on that I don't like but I can't say, because I'm not a part of it and I didn't go and sit behind where all those Sun Dance women sit, because I'm not ready for that kind of life yet. But there's fighting, and showing off; things that I don't like.

Jackie goes on to discuss how she has learned to "detach" from other people's negative emotional states through Twelve Step recovery, rather than affirming and intensifying them. She thereby posits an authentic "traditional way" that should be followed, and uses Twelve Step–influenced ideas to argue that some people who claim to follow it are actually engaged in emotionally unhealthy behaviors.

Jackie's critique of power politics ("showing off") in contemporary spiritual practices, and praise of her uncle's emotional equanimity, echoes themes from older women's narratives. Her view that she should avoid participating in other people's problems, although couched in the Twelve Step term of "detachment," is also reminiscent of the value that older women placed on avoiding social conflict. Jackie also acknowledges that her own lack of ritual experience limits her authority to speak about contemporary spiritual practices. This assertion is interestingly contradicted, however, by the fact that even though she "can't say" all that she might, she nonetheless voices clear criticisms. Jackie's comments recognize and derive moral authority from multiple and competing rhetorical frameworks.

Through both their discourse and practice, then, younger women challenge locally conventionalized ways of reckoning social identity and political authority. In so doing, they have sparked both support and criticism from other community members at Northern Cheyenne.

Since the 1980s, younger women's growing participation in ritual practices has accompanied new degrees and forms of involvement in other social arenas on the reservation, such as tribal government. Many of the most visible figures in these efforts have been women involved in recovery. The controversies surrounding their activities reflect a number of broader debates in the community that previous chapters describe. Controversy has accompanied changing gender roles and has intensified with women's rising economic power since the 1970s. The arena of ritual practice is also a site of considerable local debate. Underwriting these conflicts are broader concerns about how to legitimate political authority, especially given how many younger women are refashioning its foundations in terms of a particular conceptualization of emotional health.

Gender Politics and Contested Rituals

Various forms of tension and conflict between genders have been documented at Northern Cheyenne since at least the 1970s. Recall that women's greater participation in the local labor market by this era marked a major departure from the past. The more frequent occurrence of domestic and sexual violence or its emergence as a subject of community commentary also seems to index changing gender roles and constructions by this era.

As numerous cross-cultural studies have demonstrated, women can often claim moral authority in both public and private arenas by referencing their social roles as caregivers. Presentations by female staff

members about codependency at Recovery Center, for example, sometimes emphasized women's roles as "life-givers" whose responsibility for
others necessitated good care for oneself as a starting point for managing the difficulties of meeting responsibilities without unduly sacrificing
one's own well-being (see also Borovoy 2005). These discussions often
highlighted how local cultural constructions of women's roles emphasize fulfilling responsibilities to others more than maintaining personal
health. Depending on who was running the session, the discussion
would either founder on these complexities or try to actively address
them. One common theme when discussions continued was what some
women felt was a misuse of claims about tradition that were made to
exclude and belittle women. Some women questioned whether such
claims accurately portrayed past practices, while others argued that even
if they did, some modification of past practices to meet new conditions
was needed anyway.

Yet Northern Cheyenne women themselves clearly articulate a number
of diverse perspectives about these topics. These debates intensify when
topics turn to ritual practices. One of the most visible revitalizations of
ritual in the latter half of the twentieth century is the greater use of sweat
lodges, but fasting and collective rituals like Sun Dance are also prominent at Northern Cheyenne. By the 1990s, a variety of younger-generation women had begun building and running their own sweat lodges,
fasting, and participating in meetings of ceremonial people to plan collective rituals. While some older women have become actively involved
in Sun Dance, fasting, and other local ritual activities, particularly after
their childbearing years, many share the view that knowledge about such
matters belongs to specialists. Vicky shares her views on the resurgence of
sweat lodges in the following conversation with me.

v: You never used to see just anybody sweat—just the medicine men,
the ones that doctored, in Birney. Just one that I knew of. I used to put
up the flaps for them, go around [inside the lodge], and then drink
water. I never did take part [in the ritual itself]. I still respect them.
People try to invite me now, but I never did take part.
e: Do you feel like people who go to sweats now are not being
respectful?
v: Oh, no. It's what they do, if they were taught or feel comfortable,
then it's what they do. I don't take part myself because that's how I
was taught.

While Vicky is not explicitly critical or claiming that such practices are creating possible harm to their participants or others here, and reiterates the theme that differences are normal and expectable in ritual practice since people do as they are taught, she does remark that these practices have changed.

Other community members define the new levels of participation in sweat lodge and other ritual activities as harmful, however, especially with respect to the involvement of women. I heard a number of men comment that in engaging with ritual practices in these new ways, women were overstepping their bounds. Some men were particularly offended that women would fast at Bear Butte, since, as one man told me, Bear Butte is where Sweet Medicine was taught and where the Sacred Arrows were given to him, and it is essentially conceptualized as a male lodge. Another society man publicly criticized women for running sweat lodges.

This politics of tradition and authenticity seems in part to be the latest in a long series of political conflicts over ritual practices on the reservation. But it may well also reflect men defending their turf. With prominent trends limiting their political and economic roles, and with an increasing disengagement from family life in at least some sectors, ritual practices constitute a venue for culturally meaningful masculine social action. Northern Cheyenne women's roles in local ritual practices seem to have become more limited through much of the early and middle twentieth century (see also Ward et al. 1995).

The localized politics surrounding younger women's growing knowledge of ritual practices are multifaceted, as demonstrated by responses to one younger-generation woman who offered public talks about Cheyenne cultural heritage. These sessions were intended to instill pride in youth and to convey how violence against women and children is antithetical to traditional Cheyenne morality. The speaker discussed events within the Sun Dance ceremony as part of this talk. She was known in the community not to be involved in Sun Dance ceremonies herself, and she freely acknowledged this fact in my handful of individual conversations with her. She saw her use of this knowledge as legitimate, however, given her broader goals—and possibly too, her awareness of the local political power and rhetorical force of ceremonial knowledge. During one of this speaker's presentations, an older woman I knew kept looking over at me. She had extensive experience with Sun Dance, fasting, and other Cheyenne ritual practices herself, and told me afterward that the information presented was inaccurate. Not only that, she continued, but she had gotten a headache from being present when specialized knowledge was being discussed inaccurately and in an inappropriate context.

Yet not all community members criticize the legitimacy of younger women's growing ritual knowledge and participation. Another older woman, whose parents were highly respected for their knowledge of Cheyenne spiritual practices, chose to complete a series of fasts to benefit her family. She selected a younger-generation woman as her instructor, positively affirming the authority of younger women's knowledge as well as the innovative involvement of women in Native spiritual pursuits.

Diverse and contradictory perspectives on younger women's authority and new forms of involvement in spiritual practices have also been visible in tribal politics. Recall that the end of the 1990s featured the election of a younger woman as the first female tribal president since this form of elected government was implemented in the 1930s. This woman was involved in the trend of women engaging in Cheyenne ritual practices. Her term in office featured strong antidrug and antialcohol policies, but also extensive debates and dissension amongst (primarily male) Tribal Council members, and a threatened impeachment that was contested in a heated community meeting. She was subsequently defeated in her bid for reelection.

While multiple factors clearly shape responses to presentations, choices of ritual instructors, and the outcomes of political elections, these brief examples document how younger women's new claims to authority are meeting with both criticism and affirmation on the reservation. Younger women's entry into new roles and activities has sparked ongoing controversy. The special appeal of the Twelve Steps to younger women may reflect an attraction to a new rhetorical tool that supports their efforts not only to construct a tenable sense of personal identity, given how their capacities to engage conventional constructions of personhood are compromised, but also to persuasively claim greater moral authority within the political landscape at Northern Cheyenne.

Evaluating legitimacy in new terms such as emotional health can directly challenge the authority of elders, however, and therefore spark intense controversy. Susan illustrates a basic generational conflict by recounting a conversation with her mother, noting how, by Twelve Step standards, the moves to protect the authority of elders sometimes seem "enabling."

When I started learning about recovery and whatnot, I realized that it was a cycle that was passed across generations. And I was visiting with my mother one day, talking about how her mother and her and me [all got involved in similar kinds of marriages], and, whoa—she got defensive, she said, "You leave my mother out of this." She was, like, "I don't want to hear it." A lot of that, I think, is traditional, a traditional way of thinking, not to say anything against [others, especially one's elders]. But it's almost enabling.

These conflicts and commentary take place not only among family members, but also in public life. Many older community members were outraged, for example, when a younger man involved in recovery publicly described how both he and his son had been molested by his father. Within a Twelve Step approach, this divulgence was intended to raise community awareness of the problem of childhood sexual abuse, and to promote the protection of children by publicly identifying those who might abuse them. Many older community members interpreted this act as profoundly disrespectful, however, serving no clear purpose other than to malign the older man's reputation.

These controversies further demonstrate how Twelve Step therapies take form in a distinctive cultural world on the Northern Cheyenne Reservation and accrue meaning in relation to it. Local practices such as participation in cultural revitalization by new community members on new terms, place this therapeutic tool squarely within the complexities of local politics of identity. Such politicized meanings and their attendant controversies need to be taken into consideration in efforts to promote sobriety. A final question remains: How and why have health services for alcohol problems on the reservation overlooked the social and psychological diversity of Northern Cheyenne community members, and the plurality of moral worlds that results?

Part III
Challenges and Possibilities for "Culturally Appropriate" Alcohol Services

In support of the potent critiques of colonialism and associated efforts to decolonize governing, justice, education, health, and other key institutions within indigenous communities, many anthropologists advocate greater self-determination as a strategy to improve the effectiveness of mental health services in these contexts (e.g., Kirmayer et al. 2000; O'Nell 2004). Yet in the 1980s and 1990s, ethnographic studies of programs for substance abuse in indigenous communities expressed criticism of how some new efforts were grounded in simplistic and essentialized understandings of Native "culture" (e.g., Brady 1995; Spicer 2001; Weibel-Orlando 1989). These studies have initiated an agenda for understanding the cultural politics that currently surround substance abuse services in indigenous communities that stands to profit from greater use of insights from current social theory.

For example, Bourdieu's formulation of practice theory emphasizes the reproduction of social hierarchies and inequalities (1990). By adapting his focus on how social positioning and subjectivity relate, developments in practice theory in psychological anthropology have offered insight into how individuals variably respond to the social locations that they occupy by virtue of social structures, current political debates, and so forth (e.g., Holland and Leander 2004). For substance abuse services, this perspective encourages attention to how service programs represent substance use as a problem within the institutional context of a particular historical moment, and how individuals involved in administering, providing, or receiving these services may variably engage and reject elements of particular therapeutic approaches.

Insights from critical medical and psychological anthropology (Lock and Scheper-Hughes 1996; Scheper-Hughes 1992) complement this version of practice theory, by foregrounding how efforts to maintain or extend political hierarchies based on class, race/ethnicity, gender, nation, or other prominent social categories can impact social positioning and subjectivity (see also M. Good et al. 2008). From this perspective, socially situated actors experience powerful external pressures, such as the political-economic power of the nation-state, that can constrain the rhetorics through which local experiences are expressed and problems defined, as well as the material resources needed to develop interventions.

Integrating these insights to examine state-funded substance abuse programs in Native North America highlights the ongoing significance of structural inequalities for substance abuse programs in these contexts. In their decades of longitudinal work about drinking and psychiatric disorders in the Navajo Reservation community, Kunitz and Levy note how "Fourth World" politics shape the incorporation of local healing modalities into federally or otherwise externally funded services, and they conclude that the need to establish "bureaucratic legitimacy" (1994:217) results in a focus on measures and record keeping that narrows and rigidifies both the conceptual and material foundations of Navajo healing. Waldram additionally identifies the problem of "scientific hegemony" (1997:207) in health care for First Nations, in which alternatives to normative Euro-Canadian ways of knowing about a problem or measuring the effectiveness of an intervention are overlooked. In her work in urban Los Angeles, Weibel-Orlando (1999) also documents how changing federal policies and funding streams can suddenly and unpredictably impact addiction services for Native Americans. Further attending to how such structural pressures influence both personal experience and localized rhetorical politics in Native North America (Csordas 1999) usefully develops these insights and can offer a richer understanding of how gaps emerge between actual local needs and available health services.

To find out more about local experiences of such gaps between health needs and resources, I conducted semistructured interviews with a range of health care staff and community leaders. Initially, I conducted several brief interviews between 1994 and 1997, then followed these with more detailed interviews in 2005 with a total of 23 people. These include approximately equal numbers of men and women who have worked in health care and/or tribal government positions for anywhere from 5 to 40 years, with the overwhelming majority having over 20 years of such experience. Many people's career trajectories have included multiple jobs in the reservation's health care system, with clinical as well as administrative and managerial positions. About half have a high school education plus additional specialized paraprofessional training in their fields, while the remainder have completed college degrees (most at an associate's or bachelor's level) and/or professional certification in their specialty. All but three are enrolled members of the Northern Cheyenne Tribe (two are members of other tribes, and one is non-Native). My findings here are also informed by participant observation within the health care system.

While my data more heavily emphasize perspectives from Tribal Health staff, they also include those of current and former staff members of the Indian Health Service. Recall that health care services on the reservation are provided by federal funding that is channeled through two institutions, Tribal Health Services and the U.S. Public Health Service's Indian Health Service. These two institutions are both centrally involved in providing local health services and have a complex relationship that features both collaboration and conflict.

7
Reservation Health Care and the Politics of Local Control

The diversity of social experiences and perspectives among Northern Cheyenne community members has produced multiple understandings of sobriety and pathways toward it. As Northern Cheyenne women's experiences demonstrate, this diversity is grounded in patterned differences in subjective experience, perception, and motivation that both shape and are shaped by the political processes that accompany efforts to define and address contemporary community problems. So how and why does the primary institutionalized program to support sobriety on the Northern Cheyenne Reservation remain oriented around the Twelve Steps, despite widespread recognition of the need for more locally culturally appropriate approaches and ongoing grassroots efforts toward alternatives?

A partial answer emerges with a closer look at the federal policies and institutions that structure reservation health services. In theory, self-determination legislation has enabled local control of health services and greater responsiveness to local needs for Native North Americans since the 1970s. In practice, however, health programs at Northern Cheyenne and elsewhere continue to face complex material and discursive barriers to fashioning localized responses to health problems. A distinctive politics of knowledge accompanies how health problems are defined and addressed within federally funded health systems in indigenous communities, authorizing some ways of thinking and talking about health problems over others and, in some cases, privileging an unduly narrow range of claims about what causes a health problem or what intervention would help to alleviate it. To date, only a handful of historical and ethnographic studies have begun to examine these issues in relation to substance abuse services (Brady 1995; Gone 2008; Kunitz and Levy 1994; Weibel-Orlando 1989) and other health programs (Davies 2001; Durie 1998; Warry 1998) within indigenous communities. Their analyses highlight the complex realities that have emerged from efforts to improve self-determination and promote decolonization in state-funded health services.

Indigenous Self-Determination and Health

The challenges of improving the local relevance of health services are certainly not unique to Northern Cheyenne. Following decades of activism for greater self-determination, a new generation of health programs in New Zealand, Canada, Australia, the United States, and elsewhere has begun to emphasize greater local control of health services in indigenous communities (Brady 1995; Davies 2001; Durie 1998; Warry 1998). The scope and consequences of such local control vary widely, however. On a material level, many programs remain partially if not fully federally funded and regulated by nonindigenous accreditation agencies (Kunitz and Levy 1994); and on an ideological level, many are structured in response to prevailing therapeutic approaches in the surrounding nonindigenous society (Gone 2008, 2009).

In the United States, local control of indigenous health services was galvanized by the 1975 Indian Self-Determination and Education Assistance Act, also known as Public Law 93-638. This legislation enabled U.S. tribes to administer individual health programs in whole or in part, essentially subcontracting federal funds for individual programs from the Indian Health Service. As such, tribes were required to provide the same services that IHS had been providing or to fill a need that IHS immediately recognized. At Northern Cheyenne, people frequently use the law's number as a verb, as in, "We 638-ed that program in the late 1980s." Health staff and community leaders report that the first program "638-ed" was a comprehensive ambulance program. Emergency medical transportation is a key service in a community with a largely rural and dispersed population, and while IHS had not been providing systematic ambulance services, they clearly recognized this need. After implementing this new program, Tribal Health then began to "638" existing programs from IHS in the 1980s and 1990s. Tribal Health initially tended to oversee more community-based health programs, while IHS continued to manage clinical services. Over time, however, Tribal Health has begun bringing an increasing number of clinical services, such as the public health nursing program and a diabetes care coordination program, under their purview.

Dissatisfied with the piecemeal nature and lack of local flexibility afforded by subcontracting individual programs from IHS, several tribes in the United States began advocating for amendments to PL 93-638. By the mid-1990s, these amendments enabled individual tribes to enter into a "model contract" with IHS, bringing all tribally run health programs under one contract. While federal authority and oversight still accompany the federal funding administered through this contract, its terms more explicitly recognize tribal rights to modify programs to better fit local needs. In theory, such a unified contract also facilitates more comprehensive local health planning than is possible with disjointed contracts for individual programs. One administrator recalled: "The best thing out of that was, you can address it to your needs, and not what Montana needs or not what this [regional IHS] area needs. It's just what your community needs are. So I think that was the best thing that could have ever happened." Her comments and the amendments themselves demonstrate that ongoing tensions surrounded the recognition of localized, community-level differences by IHS, as self-determination has been implemented in practice.

Along with many tribes, Northern Cheyenne Tribal Health has chosen to remain in a model contract with IHS. A number of other tribes have elected to go a step further into full self-governance (Adams 2000; Noren et al. 1998). Self-governance tribes essentially bypass IHS as an intermediary altogether and negotiate directly with the federal government for health care funds. The route of self-governance is advocated by some but criticized by others at Northern Cheyenne—a debate that reflects many of the key local political dynamics and associated rhetorics described throughout this book, but which bears special relevance to the question of how to improve the cultural appropriateness of reservation health services.

While the original "638" contracts, the amended model contract, and self-governance cast the relationship between tribes and IHS in significantly different terms, all three scenarios rely on federal funding for health services. As such, in all three, tribal authority over health programs remains contingent upon meeting standards set by federal agencies. Tribes can therefore most easily contract a project, program, or service system if they can demonstrate that they can administer it "as well as" the federal government can. This practical exigency promotes a tendency to default to conventional American diagnostic tools, therapeutic paradigms, and service systems, despite the fact that their cross-cultural validity and applicability is often questionable. While it is possible to make a case for diverging from these standards, doing so requires not only extra effort but also persuasively engaging the medico-scientific and bureaucratic rhetorics that legitimate such claims in federal agencies. Yet these rhetorics frequently posit essentializing understandings of cultural difference, obscuring local realities of multiplicity and diversity in indigenous communities. Ethnographic research can offer an alternative perspective.

Tribal Health Services: Self-Determination in Practice

Health staff and community leaders at Northern Cheyenne broadly share the goal of developing more locally appropriate services. All describe the need to improve the quality of services, identifying widespread problems of insufficient funding and ineffective communication as fundamental barriers. As William (a health administrator) comments, the general impoverishment of the community remains a central threat to health: "Really, I think, is the root of a lot of problems, is the lack of an economic, self-sustained community . . . unemployment at 70 percent, you know, lack of housing, lack of jobs." He and others note how provision of quality health care is also impacted by limited economic resources, since it is difficult to recruit and retain staff, given the reservation's inability to offer competitive salaries for many positions (see also Davies 2001; Jones 2004). Health care staff and community leaders also recurrently describe how many community members seek health care from the local service system but do not receive information about their health conditions or therapeutic interventions in ways that they can understand or effectively implement. Language barriers to communication are clearest for elders, many of whom did not encounter English until they first attended grade school, and who still use Cheyenne considerably in their daily lives. Yet health care staff also stress how information is simply more meaningful and better retained when communicated in Cheyenne to many other community members, who may be fully bilingual or who may understand Cheyenne well even if they do not speak it fully or regularly. From this perspective, the Cheyenne language possesses a privileged capacity to express caring and aid.

Staff clearly express how problems that undermine effective rapport between service providers and community members extend beyond language barriers, however. Medical anthropologists frequently understand healing as a positive reorientation of the experience and representation of self (Csordas and Kleinman 1996) and note how healers can facilitate or inhibit such therapeutic transformations to the extent that they establish rapport with patients and persuasively engage them in a shared narrative of positive change. Examples of failures of rapport in reservation health care were frequently raised in my interviews with health staff and community leaders as well as in daily conversations at Northern Cheyenne, however. Stories of inattentive and perfunctory care figure prominently, with examples including patients being misdiagnosed, patients with chronic conditions not being informed about the results of ongoing lab work but then being confronted once their health had reached a crisis point, and patients feeling alienated from future care after experiencing disturbing side effects of procedures (e.g., bleeding after a Pap smear) that were not adequately explained to them. Problems with well-intentioned providers lacking knowledge about the living conditions and resources available to community members are also common, leading to misunderstandings such as use of expired medications or poorly framed health education efforts that leave community members feeling threatened and alienated rather than informed and motivated.

Stories of community members and staff themselves encountering unfriendly and disrespectful attitudes among some service providers and support staff in the health care system are also widespread. Many interviewees attribute such attitudes to factors ranging from outright racism to lack of familiarity with the community among some non-Native staff. Some noted that Cheyenne staff contributed also, however, due to inappropriate distraction from work by personal problems. These different views further reflect the ongoing interplay of distinct explanations for contemporary problems on the reservation.

Despite these differences, however, health care staff and community leaders generally affirm that many community members feel profoundly dehumanized in their encounters with the reservation's health care system, perceiving themselves as being treated "like animals" (and in keeping with the Montana rangeland surrounding us, often more specifically "like cattle"). Most express that shifting the prevailing political dominance of non-Cheyennes in reservation health care by empowering community members would help to resolve these problems.

For example, most express support for training and hiring more tribal members into the health care system as a means of helping to reduce communication barriers and improve the quality of services. A number explicitly relate problems in the actions and interactions of key players in reservation health care (Tribal Health, IHS, tribal government, and community members) to legacies of oppression, and advocate for psychological and social change to resolve these problems as part of a broader process of political empowerment. Some add that a clear tribal preference in hiring helps to promote such empowerment by inspiring positive motivation in youth. Marcy (a health administrator) says, "If they knew something like that was available, you know, they'd be more willing to go into training and come back and work for the tribe. I think that's what a lot of them like to do."

Within these general points of consensus about needs and strategies for reducing cultural barriers to effective health care, health staff and community leaders also articulate several specific challenges that they face in replacing federal control of health services with substantive local control. Many portray the application of accreditation standards and limitations in reservation infrastructure as key problems. These ongoing challenges to local control of health care at Northern Cheyenne have converged especially forcefully at Recovery Center.

Recall how efforts to address alcohol in reservation health care have been shaped by changing federal policies. Initially piecemeal services were followed by a greater investment of funds and increasing pressures toward professionalization, including training and certification by external agencies. Recovery Center's current form took shape in the 1980s, with diagnostic procedures and program content based on a combination of psychiatric criteria (from the *Diagnostic and Statistical Manual of Mental Disorders*), American Society of Addiction Medicine standards, and, most centrally, Twelve Step approaches.

This professionalization process was accompanied by accreditation by external agencies, certification of counselors, and other elements associated with achieving bureaucratic legitimacy in U.S. health care. In many respects, these changes have led to enhanced resources, such as the ability to bill private insurance programs and a wider array of federal funding sources for services. Yet, as elsewhere, these same features have also produced the potential for severe and sudden resource reductions that are beyond local control. By the late 1990s, this potential had become a reality for Recovery Center.

The Challenge of Accreditation

Counseling staff at the Recovery Center were required to achieve accreditation through the regional Northwest Indian Council on Chemical Dependency in the 1980s, and by the more stringent standards of a state chemical dependency certification program by the mid-1990s. The program itself also earned accreditation through CARF (Committee on Accreditation of Rehabilitation Facilities). Yet from the accounts of Tribal Health staff, a 1997 site visit to review Recovery Center's accreditation status proved disastrous. A fire had just destroyed the IHS clinic, and Tribal Health programs were scrambling to relocate, as their space was donated to support an immediate reestablishment of IHS clinical services. Despite staff efforts to explain that these were not normal conditions, evaluators concluded that Recovery Center did not have adequate physical facilities, and the program lost its full accreditation. Budget cuts and problems with retaining and recruiting staff soon followed, and the program was rapidly and severely downsized. Its space problems were quickly resolved through relocation to a nearby trailer, and a return to its original building within two years. By summer 2005, however, Recovery Center had been without a permanent director for several years.

From the perspectives of many at Tribal Health, Recovery Center has been caught in a vicious cycle through its dependence on accreditation standards. Being held accountable to these standards exposed the fragility of its economic and human resources in ways that, to many involved in the process, seemed excessively harsh. A temporary problem with physical space resulted in the program's accreditation being made provisional, with the apparent intent that it would be fully reestablished once the program resolved the problem. But in practice, the inability to fully bill for services quickly led to a decline in economic resources, which resulted in layoffs of some staff, and the instability of the program led to the departures of others—including key managerial staff. This rapid depletion of Recovery Center's human resources does not seem to have been intended or anticipated by the accreditation agency, yet, as a result, the program faces a much larger obstacle to regaining accreditation than it did at the time of the site visit.

This experience raises thorny questions about the extent to which accreditation standards in U.S. health care should be uniform, to ensure equal quality, or flexible, to acknowledge the different resource scenarios that localized communities experience. In her widely read account of the cultural clash between well-intentioned pediatricians and caring Hmong parents in managing a severe case of epilepsy in a child in Merced, California, author Anne Fadiman (1997) emphasizes how a well-intentioned devotion to ideals of equality that translate into "sameness," rather than being accommodating and responsive to cultural difference, can undermine effective health care. Nonetheless, such standardization efforts are clearly evident in Recovery Center's accreditation experiences. These events have posed significant challenges for the program, and both its staff members and other staff in Tribal Health note how Recovery Center has been forced to divert time and energy to crisis management rather than to program development and planning. This fact alone may significantly contribute to the program's continuing reliance on Twelve Step approaches.

The fragility of the economic and human resources at Recovery Center arguably also reflects a long-standing legacy of underfunding and underdeveloped infrastructure for education and governance at Northern Cheyenne and many other Native American reservations. These legacies were widely discussed in my interviews with health staff and community leaders and also seem to have contributed to Recovery Center's inability to consistently meet conventional standards for accreditation.

The Challenge of Limited Resources

Schools on the reservation have experienced chronic under-resourcing, difficulties with recruiting and retaining staff, management problems, and high dropout rates in recent generations (Ward 2005). The local tribal community college, Chief Dull Knife College, is a key resource that provides a successful adult education program (for high school equivalency or G.E.D. completion), two-year associate's degrees, some distance-learning opportunities, and guidance to students who wish to transfer to four-year institutions off the reservation. For over a decade in the 1980s and 1990s, the college also provided a specialized program in chemical dependency counseling education, and by the mid-1990s the majority of Recovery Center staff had completed training there. Within two years of Recovery Center losing its full accreditation, however, this counselor training program also ceased operation, as its founder and director left the reservation. This event exacerbated the program's problems with recruiting new staff. Yet health care staff and community leaders report that while problems with recruiting staff may be particularly intense for Recovery Center, they are widespread across reservation health programs.

William (health administrator) links the limitations of local educational resources with a troubling dependence on outsiders to fill key positions: "We also need a more educated workforce. . . . You know, we're lacking [people with specialized clinical and public health training], and in order to get those people, we have to recruit people from way out there. And we don't have housing available for them. And we live so far out in the sticks, and maybe they like to eat Chinese or something like that—we don't have nothing like that." Others report difficulty with not only recruiting but also retaining such staff. High rates of turnover in many staff positions complicate the ability of both Tribal Health and IHS to provide consistent and comprehensive orientations to new employees in the health care system, contributing to the quality-of-care problems noted above.

Many also note problems with local governmental systems. The elected tribal president and Tribal Council members help to appoint boards that oversee key tribal functions, including Tribal Health Services. William notes a fundamental link between the economic fragility and marginality of the reservation and its systems of government, commenting, "We don't have the basic structure, governmental structure, to have a healthy, economically self-sustaining community." In his view, insufficient systems of governance facilitate the economic problems that impact the community's health and health care system (see also Cornell and Kalt 1992). Elizabeth (health support staff) describes this problem as one of instability, given how radically entire agendas for health care, economic projects, and other tribal functions can shift, from one administration to the next: "To me, it's just like it's something temporary, and then the [tribal] administration changes, and you don't know what they're going to do or what they're going to change."[1]

William, Elizabeth, and all other health care staff and community leaders that I interviewed also describe problems with the decision-making processes that characterize current governmental systems. Numerous stories depict how people in these positions sometimes make decisions based on impressionistic information drawn from their own experiences or those of their relatives. Interviewees particularly emphasize how lingering resentment over such experiences could lead elected and appointed officials to micromanage health programs, moving to cut funding to particular programs or to fire particular staff members. There is no clear infrastructure in the tribe's political system for appealing such actions, contributing to an ethos of fear and anxiety among health staff in eras in which they take place. William offers a psychological interpretation of how some community leaders "use their positions to get back at people."

> They don't know how to trust, they don't know how to respect a person, they don't know how to utilize people's talents for the greater good. And that's our major stumbling block. . . . Anything that the tribe has ever tried to operate like an enterprise, like a tribal enterprise, a lot of them fail because there's a lot of jealousy, you know. And I think that's what defeats us most, is our own dysfunctionalism. We're self-defeating, you know, we don't know how to help each other any more. We don't know how to help ourselves anymore.

Others echo these themes, including William's use of terms ("dysfunction") and concepts from Twelve Step and other popular psychology trends. Herbert (health administrator) describes the psychological dynamics of "oppression" as producing "people that are very angry and not knowing what they are angry about, [they] don't want to hear and don't want to see" anything other than their own immediate experiences. These sensibilities run counter to the careful needs assessment, long-term planning, and general stability within programs that most health staff and community leaders highlight as essential foundations for quality and locally responsive health care. As described above, this critical rhetoric about how some Cheyennes have internalized unhealthy emotional lives and motivations as a result of collective experiences of disenfranchisement is often used as a call to action in local discourse about community problems. William, Herbert, and others seem to use it in this way here, that is, not as commentary on the inevitability or hopelessness of this situation, but rather as an effort to promote positive change.

Some claim that these revenge politics are particularly intense for Recovery Center. Angela (health administrator) recalls feeling exasperated when the first meeting of a new health board started with attacks on Recovery Center, with a new elected official saying, "Well, my relative was—didn't get no help, came down here." Angela adds that since "almost the entire reservation is affected by you know, drugs, alcohol, whatever," Recovery Center may be especially subject to encountering anger, resentment, and other unresolved emotional pain that people "carry around" in relation to substance use. A number of current and former staff members of Recovery Center echo these perceptions.

Similar psychological analyses permeate commentary by health staff and community leaders about relationships among different reservation health care programs. Many describe difficulties with collaboration. As William remarks,

> We have all kinds of programs, but they all have different strategic goals and objectives. And they're all going in different directions, they're not going in a concerted effort, you know. . . . We're trying to eliminate alcoholism and drug abuse, but we need to partner with Social Services, with the judicial system, with law enforcement, with the youth clubs—you know, all of that. The system doesn't allow us to do that. We don't have the same goal in mind.

While William attributes the source of this problem to "the system," Joe (health administrator) interprets some reservation health staff's "territorial" attitudes and unwillingness to work with other programs as legacies of dependency in reservation history, which through their effects on families have fundamentally altered how Cheyennes relate to one another. In his view, "dysfunctional families" raise people who can't work together, and who too easily lose sight of common goals. An interplay of rhetorics that emphasize structural violence and those that stress more psychologically oriented perspectives on Cheyenne responsibility and agency in local social life are visible here.

Others similarly note that a lack of collaboration characterizes many health programs on the reservation. In previous years, however, I directly witnessed how Recovery Center was actively working in collaboration with the types of programs that William mentioned above. When I mentioned this, William and others attributed this fact to the staff members who were present at that time. Stories of how other health programs functioned differently depending on who staffed and/or managed them formed a frequent theme throughout many of the interviews. The fact that situations change so readily depending on the individuals involved seems further testament to a lack of stable infrastructure in the reservation's health care system.

Interviewees also describe how limited infrastructure ultimately serves to reproduce dependency on federal funds. As Elizabeth (health support staff) notes, federal priorities can change: "But you know with a war going on, you know we don't—things could change, the funding or . . . I think the tribe needs to have some grant writers. There's a lot of grants out there, they just need to—someone needs to write them. That's what we're lacking." Yet writing grants is contingent upon a final challenge of reservation infrastructure noted by several interviewees, namely, the capacity to gather and analyze the kind of data about health that are considered to be persuasive by federal and other funding agencies.

Federal funding requirements like GASB-34 (the 1999 version of standards produced by the Governmental Accounting Standards Board) emphasize that health programs must have clearly stated goals and objectives that are explicitly grounded in data. Yet resources for gathering and analyzing highly localized information about health historically have been lacking in the Indian Health Service. Instead, since its founding in the 1950s, IHS has emphasized regional area offices rather than local service units in its data collection and reporting, which generalize across numerous tribal groups and geographic areas. Staff involved in planning at Northern Cheyenne report that limited resources at IHS in recent years have also led to an emphasis on descriptive information rather than detailed analysis of the kinds of local meanings, causal associations, and so forth that are needed to persuasively document how local realities may differ from conventionalized U.S. standards.

Administrative staff also emphasize that they do not have sufficient local infrastructure for gathering and analyzing such information. One administrator demonstrated this problem by describing how he first has to go to specific programs and request information. He then showed me handwritten notes of numbers of people seeking help for a particular type of problem, noting how staff members are sometimes able to provide him with only this kind of information. He then needs to compile the information into a spreadsheet and analyze it to make use of it in the types of reports and plans that federal agencies require. While efforts are currently under way to develop more routinized information gathering and reporting strategies for Tribal Health as well as other tribal programs at Northern Cheyenne, all involved recognize the difficulties of locating appropriate human and technological resources for this undertaking.

The questions of what information to gather and how to effectively ascertain it also remain unanswered. Since most health staff recognize Northern Cheyenne as "culturally distinct" relative to other U.S. communities, their understandings about what exactly constitutes "culturally appropriate" health care are centrally at stake in any plans to improve the responsiveness of health care services to local needs. Health staff and community leaders express divergent understandings here, in ways that reflect the ongoing interplay of local interpretative frameworks and rhetorical tools for understanding community problems on the reservation. Their commentary also illuminates how federal institutional structures like accreditation and funding standards can impose both discursive and material pressures that constrain discussion about the cultural contextualization of health needs. Different perspectives among health care staff and community leaders about the meaning of local control of health services illustrate these dynamics.

The Challenge of Defining Local Control

While all health care staff and community leaders that I interviewed expressed generalized support for greater local control of health services, people differed in their perspectives on how the tribe has "638-ed" more health services during the past decade—and even more so, on the possibility of implementing full self-governance. Opinions vary widely as to whether programs contracted by Tribal Health are more responsive to community needs, better managed, or otherwise improved. Moreover, some people report growing collaboration between Tribal Health and IHS programs, while others emphasize increasing tension. For example, some counselors at Recovery Center reported in 2005 that they were effectively exchanging client referrals with emergency room, general medicine, and behavioral health components of the IHS clinic. Yet accounts of the extent of collaboration vary by programs, by individual staff members, and also across time.

Many long-term health staff describe how there can be fundamental differences in the priorities of the more clinically oriented IHS and the community health–oriented Tribal Health. Staff in both institutions describe how Tribal Health efforts to develop the field-based and outreach components of health programs have met with resistance from IHS, which focuses on the provision of services at the clinic. Angela, a longtime Tribal Health administrator, describes how with the model contract after the mid-1990s, "there are a lot more restrictions that they could not put on anymore. And they were so not used to it! It was like, it was really difficult to work with them." She notes how Tribal Health staff ultimately sought legal aid, to clearly and persuasively document their right to prioritize outreach and avoid continually expending resources to respond to resistance from IHS.

While health staff and community leaders generally agree that some degree of "638-ing" is beneficial, proponents of full self-governance currently seem to be in the minority at Northern Cheyenne. Most describe how the difficulties that Tribal Health has encountered with IHS during the model contract process have galvanized local anxieties about self-governance. For example, they note how IHS staff became convinced that their jobs would be taken away if the tribe took over administration of the clinic, with high-level clinicians even threatening to quit if self-governance were implemented. Some note how rumors circulate about how other self-governance tribes have catastrophically lost staff or are facing bankruptcy, when these claims are not true. The prominence of these anxieties suggests that leadership and support for self-governance are relatively limited.

Indeed, most people that I interviewed do not support self-governance. Joe expresses doubts by describing that some "638-ed" programs are not being managed well. Here he offers the same historical and psychological argument about the origins of behavior in families that he employed when describing other problematic actions by health employees: "You know, [through colonization and forced assimilation] we did such a good job taking responsibility away from our Cheyenne people. In our 638 programs, now we're running out of funds, and we're trying to get that responsibility back. And it's hard." Joe situates a lack of managerial skill as a consequence of the local collective history of colonization. He presents the decay of responsibility as a lengthy process that is now deeply rooted in the socialization of many Cheyenne community members, which will take time to rectify.

Similarly, Herbert identifies lack of responsibility as a key problem area, describing how the concept of self-governance initially appealed to him, but that he subsequently came to question the motives involved and now feels more comfortable with collaboration, rather than competition, between Tribal Health and IHS. He expresses ongoing mixed feelings, saying he feels that Tribal Health and IHS "can work together effectively without that institutional division. I don't know what I feel about it. I realized that it [collaboration] could work, but I wasn't giving it a chance. . . . I know it can work, without having to go to the extreme of self-governance or 638-ing everything." He grounds his concern in his own perception of a widespread lack of professionalism among health care staff whose primary work experience has been on the reservation.

> People spend a lot of time on their personal family issues or whatever, own issues at work, than they do actually doing their own work— their job that they're hired to do. It's—if anything, if we go self-governance or 638 everything, that would be our downfall right there. It's because we're going to put people in responsible positions like a clinic to serve and care for our people, and if you take as many holidays as we have, and take half days off, and come to work when we want to, and do all our own personal business on work time, we're going to run ourselves into the ground, and we'll fail. And that's not just with Indian Health Service, but with any business that we take on.

Taken alone, Herbert's statement here could be read as a disturbing recapitulation of colonial narratives about the irresponsibility and immaturity of Native people or their inability to function within modern institutions. Yet Herbert avoids essentializing characterizations by describing how context is the source of these problems, noting that Cheyennes or anyone else who has experience working in more structured environments develops the professional skills that those contexts require. For him, these professional standards are a high priority for major business and managerial enterprises that he feels is not widely shared by others in the community.

Other interviewees voice similar perspectives about how the cultural context and social dynamics of reservation life are fundamentally not compatible with the functions necessary for such enterprises (see also Cornell and Kalt 1992). The local importance of kinship ties figures prominently in their accounts, which often conclude with the assertion that the community simply "isn't ready" to take on these types of enterprises. As Joe expresses:

> We're related to everybody, our services reflect that. The relatives get all the good things. . . . Indian people, on their own reservations, just aren't business-minded. There's too much—too many relatives and too much politics involved. . . . Let's just, let them—bring them in to help us. I think then they could see it in a different way. Because we're only seeing it one way, and we need somebody else's perspective. . . . So I

> would just as soon that self-governance be forgotten, you know. . . .
> We're not ready, we're not business people, we're just not ready for it.

Marcy weaves concerns about governmental stability into a similar account of kinship politics, in her critique of self-governance.

> Well, you know, I was always against self-governance. I was—I really didn't want it to happen. 'Cause I thought we weren't ready. And look what happened, you know, this new [tribal] administration came in, and it's completely different. . . . Complete turnaround, and that would have been disastrous for us, I think, if we had gone into self-governance. . . . My way of thinking is if we're going to start something big, I always think it's better to have somebody come in from the outside and run it. Manage it. And teach somebody to manage it. Because we've had some businesses where, you know, our own tribal people, tribal members have tried to run it, and it didn't work. It's too much, you know. Politics get involved. And then the tribal member will hire all their own family, and, you know, without any kind of qualifications. And it hits bottom, doesn't work. And, you know, I've seen a lot of that happen, and that's my belief, is just to hire somebody from the outside that's, you know, it doesn't matter if they're Caucasian or Indian. Somebody that has the skills to do it. And let them run it for a while. Show our people what to do. And be fair to everybody! That's what I'd like to see happen.

The accounts of proponents and critics of self-governance seem to highlight ongoing debates on the reservation about whether local cultural practices and values can really be effectively integrated with the standards of large-scale bureaucratic organization. They cast important local realities like kinship responsibilities as fundamentally in tension with the principles of fairness that are needed to make such institutions work effectively.

In lieu of supporting self-governance, most health care staff and community leaders that I interviewed express a sense that both Tribal Health and IHS already exist, are both working on the same problems, and both face the same issues of limited funding—so, they might as well work together. From their perspectives, the reasons for undertaking such a radical and time-, energy-, and resource-consuming change to achieve more tribal control were simply not persuasive. Some note that there were benefits to continuing fuller collaboration with IHS. For example, Andy (health administrator) notes how the national structure of the IHS enabled them to seek funds to help to cover cost overruns, whereas a contract is set in terms of its finances, and a tribe alone is far less able to access additional financial resources. Others question the motives underwriting efforts to gain greater local control. Meredith (health administrator) comments: "I think we need to network together. We all deal with same clients, same patients. And we need to stay together. That way they'll be better serviced." To her, the major motivations behind the movement toward self-governance seem negative rather than constructive: "There's a lot of people that are still prejudiced out there. They don't like doctors, they don't like nurses, they don't like—you know, like that . . . . And it's just a personal issue, you know." Others offer a more pragmatic logic, like Maria (community leader), who articulates both the pros and cons of institutionalizing greater tribal control and concludes that both Tribal Health and IHS offer different strengths. Since even self-governance is not going to remove the influence of the federal government, she reasons, continuing with the more balanced collaboration facilitated by the model contract makes the most sense.

The differences in perspectives and priorities visible in the debates over how (and more specifically, how much) to institutionally implement greater local control of health services highlight the interplay of distinct local rhetorics for characterizing the conditions of reservation life. Some people prioritize freedom from the constraints imposed by IHS as an essential means to achieving better health care, highlighting undue external pressures and controls over reservation life. Others cast localized cultural priorities as incompatible with the managerial functions required by large-scale enterprises or question the need for what they view as radical and rapid change. Some specifically question the motives behind institutionalizing greater local control, offering historical and psychological characterizations of the legacies of colonization in support of their claims. These differences illustrate the divergent meanings that health staff and community leaders attribute to "local control" of health services. More broadly, they also demonstrate the complex rhetorical politics that can accompany these diverse perspectives and priorities on the reservation. While this diversity is widely evidenced in community life, it is frequently overlooked when discussions explicitly turn to strategies for providing more culturally appropriate health services.

The Challenge of Defining Culturally Appropriate Services

From an anthropological perspective, culture consists of a repertoire of ideas and patterns of social organization that shape experience, perception, and motivation. It is often characteristic of a community defined by past or present geographic ties but can also characterize other social groups produced by shared interests or activities. Contemporary understandings accommodate diversity and debate among members of cultural communities, as well as processes of historical change (e.g., Herzfeld 1997; Ortner 2006). Medical and psychological anthropologists also focus on the political dimensions of cultural influence on human experience and have attended especially to the impact of power inequalities on experiences of sickness, suffering, and healing. Many have highlighted how the narrowing of rhetorical frameworks for representing such experiences can serve to both obfuscate and reproduce the origins of social inequalities (e.g., Farmer 1999; Lock and Scheper-Hughes 1996; Scheper-Hughes 1992).

Understandings of culture outside of anthropology are often more static and monolithic, however, relying on essentializing logics rather than acknowledging diversity and change. As discussed above, for example, at Northern Cheyenne as in other contemporary Native North American communities (Dole and Csordas 2003; O'Nell 1996), culture is often understood in terms of "tradition." Community members who do not speak Cheyenne, engage in ceremonial practices, or have detailed knowledge of Cheyenne folklore and historical narratives sometimes present themselves as "less cultural" than those who do. Mike (health administrator) comments in discussing the need to develop more culturally appropriate health programs: "I really don't know. 'Cause it's sad— *I'm not a tribal cultural person.* I grew up here, I'm enrolled here, I can understand a few words, but I am not a fluent language speaker. . . . But I think we all have a responsibility to try and keep some of that intact" (emphasis added). He describes feeling a responsibility to maintain language and other "tribal cultural" features, but not feeling that he himself is a true participant in this world. From an anthropological perspective, however, these perceptions and distinctions are themselves part of the repertoire of ideas that constitute the local cultural landscape of reservation life. To equate "tradition" with "culture," and to understand the meanings of either/both as fixed rather than subject to ongoing social negotiation, is to engage in a historically situated cultural politics with consequences that warrant examination.

As discussed throughout the preceding chapters, such claims can enact current local power inequalities but can also be formulated to challenge them. Essentializing constructions of tradition in part offer a moral commentary that affirms positive differences between Cheyenne and non-Native worlds. Yet when cast in rigid and exclusive terms, they also underwrite the local political authority of those who can persuasively claim to be traditional over those who cannot. Efforts to improve the cultural appropriateness of health services that equate culture with tradition inevitably encounter these localized politics.

Yet institutional requirements for consistent and standardized procedures also work to privilege the idea that tradition is a clear and stable object, rather than a polysemic and fluid discursive arena. The untenability of these simplistic characterizations of complex local realities contributes to the difficulties that Recovery Center staff face in developing and implementing programs that utilize local spiritual leaders and activities (e.g., the Traditional Component, see chapter 3), and to the ongoing tendency for Recovery Center's services to remain organized around Twelve Step approaches.

Counseling staff certainly recognize the insufficiencies of Recovery Center's approaches. Some pragmatically offer local alternatives to standard Twelve Step practices, albeit in an ad hoc fashion. As one counselor describes, she allows interested clients to substitute attendance at sweat lodges and sober activities like powwows, or visits to sober relatives (especially elders), for group meetings and educational sessions at Recovery Center. She meets with them weekly at first and then monthly as they establish a new set of activities that support their sobriety. Another counselor treats exercise classes and other health-promoting activities as allowable substitutes for her clients. These modifications have elicited criticism from other health staff, however.

For example, Mike (health administrator) characterizes Recovery Center as follows: "The problem here is that there's no standardization, everybody's kind of doing their own thing the way they think it should be done, they're not following the Twelve Step model." Here he portrays individualized services as chaotic, and privileges the consistent use of one conventional therapeutic approach. His perspectives do not explicitly oppose the recognition of diversity among clients or the development of locally grounded, individualized services whose foundations are

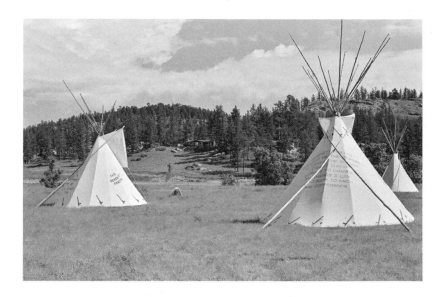

Figure 6. These tipis, erected on the powwow grounds south of Lame Deer for a 1997 intertribal sobriety campout hosted by Northern Cheyenne Tribal Health, are printed with the serenity prayer commonly used in A.A. meetings: "God grant me the serenity to accept the things I cannot change, courage to change the things I can, and wisdom to know the difference." Photo by the author.

clearly documented (rather than determined on an unclear basis by individual counselors). But they do attest to the importance of standardization among many local health staff and among higher-level administrators especially, who experience and encounter these requirements on a daily basis when interacting with federal agencies.

Instead of formally incorporating traditional or other alternative therapies, many new program developments at Recovery Center have focused on making Twelve Step concepts and practices more intelligible to community members. As one counselor described,

> There are a lot of people out there we don't even reach, who don't even know about the program. Like people who are on the streets, we get them into the process but they don't really—they go to treatment but they don't seem to get much out of it. Our treatment centers are really designed for English-speaking people, for one thing. Because if you sit down with somebody that spoke Cheyenne as a little kid, and say,

"What do you think about denial?" they don't have a clue, what denial is, you know. Or you show them a video, and nobody says anything. The only way to really explain it is to say, "OK here, here's what I did, here's how I was denying my problem," you know.

Thus, while Recovery Center staff members frequently agree with the need for a more flexible and locally relevant approach to promoting sobriety, an emphasis on a person's desire to change has remained a prominent foundation for their services. To move beyond this framework and effectively accommodate diverse local perspectives on the self-transformation of sobriety would first involve characterizing the competing and sometimes contradictory understandings and expectations among community members. Such an undertaking would be difficult and time-consuming under the best of conditions, and has been impossible, given the institutional instability recently experienced by Recovery Center. If accomplished, this characterization and the resulting need to institutionalize diverse pathways toward sobriety and individualized care plans would also need to be communicated to federal agencies. But as described above, institutional requirements continue to emphasize the standardization of services.

In these ways, Northern Cheyenne experiences with alcohol services highlight how the political power of funding sources and accreditation agencies can impact local interpretations of health problems, as well as the broader problem of how limited financial and human resources impact local infrastructures for developing and administering health programs. While these structural pressures have clearly contributed to the entrenchment of a Twelve Step approach at Recovery Center, their causal role is sometimes indirect. Accreditation standards do not explicitly dictate that Recovery Center use therapeutic approaches that have been conventionalized within alcohol treatment in the non-Native United States, for example, but they do require a clear explanation of the rationale, scope, and consequences of a culturally appropriate therapeutic approach. In practice, this combination of divergent local interpretations of sobriety, the politics that surround cultural identity and social authority, and structural pressures that do not support the capacity of service systems to respond to these complexities all work to complicate local capacities to meet these standards of clarity and coherence.

What has resulted at Northern Cheyenne during the period of my study are alcohol recovery services that are oriented by default around the Twelve Steps and that often fit poorly with local needs. The various ad hoc strategies implemented by Recovery Center staff and the grassroots activities of community members described in preceding chapters reflect ongoing local efforts to create more culturally appropriate support systems for sobriety.

8
Concluding Thoughts

Institutionalized health services to address alcohol-related problems on the Northern Cheyenne Reservation face a distinctive set of challenges. The complexities of the local cultural environment, coupled with the political-economic marginalization of this Native American community work to limit resources for developing and implementing programs that can respond effectively to the multiple and contested local meanings of sobriety. From an anthropological perspective, the local history and patterning of this diversity and debate are what make Northern Cheyenne a culturally distinctive community. Appreciating this perspective on "culture" seems an essential first step toward developing more culturally appropriate resources to support sobriety on the reservation.

My findings especially emphasize the psychological and social significance that various approaches to sobriety hold for different community members, and therefore challenge "one size fits all" types of alcohol services. Openly recognizing multiple alternatives appreciates and accepts the social and psychological diversity among community members, rather than imposing a universalized approach that can help only those who accept it or are willing and able to modify it. Better understandings of the local social arenas that are psychologically salient for community members, and of the consequences of switching from drinking to sobriety within those arenas, are needed to clarify how well and for whom particular therapeutic approaches might hold the greatest appeal. Evaluating the effectiveness of specific therapies, while an important and pressing need, cannot be fully accomplished without understanding these local cultural complexities.

Ethnographic research about substance abuse in Native North America is well positioned to further examine such cultural complexities. Recent research and commentary by ethnographers including Weibel-Orlando (1989), Brady (1995), Spicer (2001), Medicine (2007), and Gone (2008) have posed preliminary answers to two vital questions: (1) how to better support sobriety in Native communities, and (2) how to effectively support greater local control of health services.

Most of these authors agree that spirituality and local ritual practices are widely recognized within Native American communities as important tools for promoting sobriety and warrant further study. Most also emphasize that better social support for sobriety appears to be the most promising mechanism for alleviating problems related to substance use, and that clearer investigations of how social dynamics (e.g., kinship, community) do and might further serve to support sobriety are needed. My findings confirm these directions for future research but also call for closer attention to how community members seeking sobriety may be situated in multiple ways within a variety of wider-ranging local debates. At Northern Cheyenne, for example, opportunities and motivations for sobriety are shaped by socially patterned and conflicting perspectives about emotional expression, self-transformation, institutional authority, inclusiveness in local spiritual traditions, and self-governance in health care.

Careful attention to how access to ritual practice and other sources of social support are shaped by these localized politics would better help those seeking sobriety to see diverse possibilities and locate those that best fit their own subjective realities. As Gone (2008) documents in a First Nations community in Northern Manitoba, eclectic services from multiple therapeutic traditions (Aboriginal, Western, Eastern) can be effectively integrated in a substance abuse program run by and for Native North Americans—and even this diversity can be integrated though a shared metaphor for healing (e.g., Medicine Wheel) that is broadly appealing to local clients yet also responsive to their diversity. In addition to undertaking such local developments of services, alcohol programs in Native communities can consider a variety of approaches developed by and for Native peoples that are circulating nationally. Modifications of Twelve Step approaches for Native North Americans that incorporate collective experiences of colonization and common conventions for social interaction are available (e.g., Coyhis and White 2002). Therapies that are grounded in the cultural heritage of specific tribes, yet potentially useful to others, are also offered (e.g., Walle 2004). Yet Northern Cheyenne experiences suggest that the preconditions necessary for implementing these approaches within federally funded health services remain highly localized and often elusive.

Better understanding of the power relations that shape health resources in specific times and places would provide a fuller assessment of whether and how indigenous communities are able to fashion substance abuse services that meet local needs. Taking cues from Csordas (1999) and O'Nell (1996) about the significance of local social arenas for identity politics in Native North America helps to illuminate how addiction/recovery therapies relate to ongoing experiences of structural violence. Local rhetorical conventions for contrasting past with present hold striking parallels to common non-Native narratives that frame all change as corruption and loss, positioning contemporary Native peoples as inherently inferior to their ancestors as well as to non-Natives. At Northern Cheyenne, younger women's reconfigurations of this rhetoric can be seen as contesting the disordering impact of colonization upon local systems of meaning. One could read their use of Twelve Step terms and concepts in this process as an imposition of non-Native ethnopsychological constructs, however. Yet the selectivity evident in how Northern Cheyenne women make use of Twelve Step approaches, along with the continuing salience of localized understandings of gender roles, emotion, spirituality, and cultural authority that are visible in local responses to the Twelve Steps, requires a more multidimensional reading of the creativity and constraints involved.

If institutionalized health services were to more fully recognize the diversity of local strategies for achieving sobriety at Northern Cheyenne, as well as the politics that surround therapeutic interventions for alcohol problems on the reservation, then the alcohol program at Northern Cheyenne would be able to invest in far more pluralism and flexibility. Ethnographic research that focuses greater attention on barriers to doing so can assist Native communities who are currently experiencing disjunctures between their mental health service systems and local community needs. In the United States, entrenched patterns of misrecognizing diversity within and among Native peoples align with broader U.S. cultural tendencies to individualize and political tendencies to privatize responsibility for health. What results are profound tendencies toward essentializing logics in understanding and addressing health problems that can be helpfully complicated by the cultural contextualization that ethnography offers.

Yet lack of recognition of ethnographic insights by federal health institutions in the United States remains an ongoing problem for Native North America (Manson 1997) and pressures tribes and community advocates to contend with overly narrow definitions of what constitutes legitimate knowledge about health. These politics of knowledge also must change if the cultural appropriateness of mental health services in Native North American communities such as Northern Cheyenne is to improve. Further research examining how funding and regulatory institutions set forth parameters for knowledge claims, and how different Native American communities have accommodated or transformed these discourses in constructing claims about their own local health experiences and needs (e.g., Kelm 2004), could offer constructive support for change.

Of course, one could also conclude that the current federally funded health service system is simply unable to respond effectively to local community needs. Along similar lines, Smith (2005) argues compellingly that the conventional justice system in the United States is so invested in reproducing troubling social inequalities that Native American communities are better off developing alternative community-based systems of restorative justice. Yet in the case of health care, moving entirely outside of the federally funded health service system raises larger ethical questions. Currently, for example, the fact that local alcohol services at Northern Cheyenne have remained centered on the Twelve Steps has essentially delegated responsibility for fashioning locally relevant services to community members themselves—and in practice, particularly to women. By simply recognizing and affirming such grassroots efforts, the federal government could engage in what looks like endorsement of Native sovereignty while essentially abrogating its responsibilities to Native peoples.

Rights to health care for the survivors of massive losses and violations of rights are expressly recognized in generations of U.S. federal policy regarding Native peoples. Even if ambivalence and ineffectiveness have too often characterized understandings of Native health problems and the resources devoted to addressing them (Jones 2006), it seems important to advocate for improvement. Numerous and detailed negotiations would need to take place to more fully reconcile federal responsibilities and funding with local needs and therapeutic resources. At Northern Cheyenne, my findings suggest that sorting through the complex politics that currently surround self-determination and self-governance, both among tribal members and between tribal institutions like Tribal Health and federal ones like the Indian Health Service, would be centrally at stake in such negotiations.

Given these complexities, while both local and federal resources are clearly available to better address alcohol problems, and multiple possibilities abound, it is difficult to discern exactly what the future holds at Northern Cheyenne. Since the 1994–2005 period of my study, there are hopeful signs that feedback is improving between Recovery Center and the ongoing grassroots efforts to improve the cultural relevance of addiction services at Northern Cheyenne. By late 2005, key Recovery Center staff were developing the kinds of culturally specific descriptions of services that meet accreditation and funding standards, such as protocols for referring interested clients to participate in sweat lodge rituals at accessible locations around the reservation. They were also working with a newly invigorated regional tribal leaders association to procure new resources for alcohol and other substance abuse services. A new director for Recovery Center was hired in 2006, and in 2009 the program itself was renamed Seven Feathers Healing Center, reflecting its investment in providing culturally appropriate services. Yet in these early stages, it is difficult to tell the extent to which these new developments are responding to the central needs highlighted in this study, such as incorporating more pluralism and flexibility in services that actively respond to the diversity of meanings and politics of practice that surround sobriety on the reservation.

By offering an ethnographically contextualized analysis of narratives produced by Northern Cheyenne women with interests in personal and/ or community alcohol problems and using these to analyze how gender, generation, and other dimensions of diversity inform how drinking and sobriety are understood and approached by Northern Cheyenne community members, my work here builds upon current efforts in anthropology to better theorize and represent the historical and cultural contextualization of subjective experience (Biehl et al. 2007; M. Good et al. 2008; Ortner 2006). In both their content and rhetorical features, narratives can offer insight into how personal experiences of suffering can shape ongoing needs for meaning that influence how people think, feel, and respond to the conditions of their lives. As people have experiences and seek to make sense of them, they navigate through culturally available interpretations and in the process may create new ones that themselves circulate in local social life, generating responses in turn. Through such circulation, these interpretations and their associated concepts, rhetorical tools, and practices themselves accrue layers of meaning that influence who uses them and how. Situating narrative analysis within broader community-based research methods like participant observation offers a means of tracking these political processes.

As a form of person-centered research, narrative analysis also offers opportunities for detailed analysis of how individuals personalize cultural resources. It has not been my goal here to analyze these processes per se; instead, my focus on the relationships between social positioning and forms of talk is driven by the larger goal of delineating patterns that need to be better understood to improve the "cultural appropriateness" of alcohol services at Northern Cheyenne. Any human community will include diverse individuals, but not all include the same degree of active reflection on what constitutes "our culture," or social patterns in how people orient themselves to these debates, that I witnessed at Northern Cheyenne. People everywhere seek resources (e.g., symbols, rituals, and so forth) from their available cultural worlds for expressing and communicating their experiences of suffering, often in a quest for therapeutically transforming such realities and finding a way to live with more peace and less pain. Yet Northern Cheyenne experiences demonstrate the layers of complexity that are introduced into these processes when social diversity is misrecognized and material resources are limited in a community.

By describing the political-economic conditions that shape how key resources for alcohol problems are used, and by documenting how local grassroots alternatives to federally funded recovery services have emerged, my findings also reflect ongoing anthropological efforts to integrate meaning-centered investigations with political-economic analyses, and further extend these efforts into ethnographic studies of sobriety in Native North America. Continuing such efforts will generate opportunities to speak to larger anthropological concerns. For example, critically evaluating concepts that figure prominently within indigenous substance abuse services, like historical trauma, stands to further refine scholarly understandings of when and how it makes sense to use psychological terms to understand collective experiences (e.g., see Gone 2009; B. Good et al. 2008).

Considering both the psychological and sociopolitical depth of localized diversity and debate about drinking and sobriety at Northern Cheyenne also affirms and extends medical anthropology's broad goals of understanding the tensions that so often arise at the interface between local cultural worlds and health services whose ideas and practices are developed or funded at national or international levels. Indeed, such tensions are widespread. The story of Northern Cheyenne experiences with alcohol services contributes to a better accounting of how alcohol treatment has emerged and evolved in the United States as well. A reliance on Twelve Step philosophies, principles, and techniques continues to be common in the United States despite considerable ongoing criticism. Critics have called for more evidence-based alternatives (cognitive-behavioral therapies, motivational interviewing, and so forth) in health programs that address substance abuse. Recent decades have also witnessed the development of a wide variety of self-help alternatives for Americans who want to change their drinking practices, including some more secular and some more explicitly religious (e.g., grounded in evangelical Christianity) than A.A.; some like Rational Recovery that focus on the shorter term as an alternative to A.A.–style ongoing participation; and some that aim for goals other than abstinence, such as controlled drinking (White 1998). While certainly different in form and degree, the focus on cultural debates and resource flows that I have described for Northern Cheyenne may be quite relevant for understanding how Twelve Step approaches are situated relative to alternatives in the United States more generally. Ongoing broader public ambivalence about whether and how alcohol use truly constitutes a health problem rather than a moral one, for example, may serve as a barrier to investments in change once particular therapeutic approaches have become conventionalized. Economics also play a role: many health programs contend with uncertain resources and limitations on recruiting and retaining staff that may also serve as such a barrier. The reasons how and why Twelve Step approaches rose to such widespread prominence in both self-help and professional treatment for alcohol and related problems in the United States, and the extent to which their prevalence is related to their effectiveness, remain intriguing empirical questions for continuing study.

With tools for examining the interplay between cultural context and subjective experience in therapeutic transformations of thought, feeling, and behavior, ethnographic research is especially well positioned to explore how Twelve Step concepts and practices are circulating in a wide variety of different cultural contexts in our contemporary world—and to enrich understanding of their intertwining psychological, social and political consequences.

Epilogue 1
Stephanie Timber (pseudonym),
Northern Cheyenne Reservation

The early chapters of this book capture the essence of the historical events that have threatened to eradicate a once strong, healthy, and independent tribal people. For the Northern Cheyenne, and most tribal peoples, a direct agent of their destruction was alcohol. The continued presence of this substance in Indian Country is unrelenting, and its consequences are devastating to health and well-being in Native communities. This agent has robbed North American Natives of their identity and traditional cultural ways as well as their authentic spiritual practices, the very core of establishing positive mental/emotional health, personal development, and productivity.

The author's knowledge of ethnographic research and style of professionalism helped her to gather qualitative in-depth personal narratives, examining the ethnopsychology of sobriety and restoration to well-being across two generations of women. From these perspectives, the author examines resilient responses to sobriety and asserts that older generations rely heavily upon returning to the moral worlds of traditional protocol and the early learning in childhood as a means to restore well-being and stop drinking. In contrast, personal narratives from the younger generation portray early childhood experiences as psychologically damaging to their well-being, and cultural and traditional protocol as nonexistent, recalling parental alcohol use and abuse as contributors to the loss of cultural identity.

The author describes a well-known alternative healing trajectory currently taking place across Indian Country today for alcohol cessation. Ethnographic findings throughout this text indicate that participating in traditional activities and traditional spirituality (sweats, Sun Dance, fasts, dance, drum, etc.) can help Northern Cheyennes to ameliorate drinking and other colonial effects. The author examines how the historically male template of traditional and spiritual practices has become an important element of resilient responses for sobriety in the younger generations.

Throughout Indian Country, claims to cultural heritage through ritual practices are noticeably recognized as essential elements to healing. Among the Northern Cheyenne, however, participation in such practices as an instrument in healing and in efforts toward a renewed personal psychological framework and spiritual connection to becoming Cheyenne is often met with controversy and criticism, with distinctively localized consequences. Despite the identity politics that result, many Northern Cheyenne have continued to pursue enculturation practices as a key component of personal health and well-being.

On the Northern Cheyenne Reservation, as well as in most Native communities, personal health and well-being are essential for our very existence. Interventions to this trajectory force us to broaden models of self-transformation that were derived from the works of past worlds into a more circumscribed context of our present world and, in doing so, enable many Northern Cheyenne to gain a renewed sense of productivity, belonging, and cultural identity. It is with this knowledge that I speak in support of the need for culturally appropriate programs to address the specific health needs in our community.

Among the Northern Cheyenne, community-based programs coordinated through self-governance are seen as both beneficial and challenging. Public Law 93-638, Indian Self-Determination and Education Act, has great potential. Imagine this: Native North Americans are the only existing people in the United States given political and economic sovereignty. In a way, this law can be seen as a gift to all North American Natives, and in a way, seen as the government's attempt to help rectify past damages.

According to my viewpoint, the ongoing collaboration between Indian Health and Tribal Health Services must integrate their services to promote quality health and well-being, while at the same time being able to objectively consider the differences between the agendas that define culturally appropriate health services in the Northern Cheyenne community. This, it seems, may mean being sensitive and responsive to, while at the same time being respectful and cognizant of, the needs of local community health programs that augment or complement both healing and reform in a culturally diverse context. Therefore, both Indian Health and Tribal Health must clearly decide their position on prevention activities and the delivering of direct services.

Self-governance is no easy task. In recent years there has been a call for greater accountability in the conduct as well as the delivery of some Tribal Health programs. Unfortunately, the dynamics of alcohol and drug use are deeply rooted in the health of our local community. Ethnographic findings in this text echo my own perspectives of key components of failure in self-governance, such as ongoing internal kinship and identity politics; community isolation; lack of technical assistance for computing and collecting data; the lack of managerial and leadership skills, technical training opportunities, professional standards in institutional structures, and ability to develop infrastructure for long-term program sustainability; and language barriers for Cheyenne-speaking elders. Proper health care on the Northern Cheyenne Reservation is contingent upon a community of healthy, professional, and spiritually developed individuals. The critical and diverse role played by local community and tribal leaders themselves and ongoing collaboration between the Indian Health and Tribal Health Services will determine whether success can be ultimately achieved in local health care.

In closing, I would like to acknowledge the author's insight, hard work, and many years of dedication to the ethnographic research presented in this text. It is my opinion that ethnographic research in Native communities includes a certain amount of personal risk. I most certainly believe, without a doubt, that Erica Prussing's trust in her own ability and strengths enabled her to encompass and express an understanding of the diverse and complex social/political structures that operate in and influence daily life on the Northern Cheyenne Reservation. Her findings are truly articulated and evidenced throughout this text.

Becoming Cheyenne is wonderful!

Epilogue 2
B. A. Brown, Northern Cheyenne Reservation

I first met Erica through a longtime friend, sociologist Carol Ward. Carol introduced me to Erica as an anthropologist who was working on her dissertation and who had arrived on the reservation to do her "fieldwork." I did not know what the field of anthropology was about or the kind of work an anthropologist did, thus my curiosity was sparked to learn more about anthropology and the type of "fieldwork" Erica would be doing.

I remember my first time sitting with Erica in the cafeteria at Dull Knife (Chief Dull Knife College), and my first question to her was to find out what kind of work she would be doing here at the reservation. The majority of my talks with Erica during her time spent here were talks centered on anthropology and its past/future direction, and her fieldwork. We shared a cultural exchange and still do.

Erica's friends at Northern Cheyenne know that she owned a big dog named Maia, who was her trusty companion while here at Northern Cheyenne. A Lab and Rottweiler mix, Maia was a huge dog with tons of energy. Maia attained celebrity status and if community members saw Erica and Maia out walking, they would jokingly tease Erica about how her huge dog was taking her for a run.

Erica would share holiday meals with my family. My mother took a liking to her immediately, and it was about a year and a half later when my mother told me that she wanted to adopt Erica as a daughter. Because Erica's demeanor brought back memories of her mother, Annie Swallow Medicinebull, at the adoption ceremony Erica would be given a Cheyenne name as well.

My brother Charles Little Old Man did the adoption ceremony at my mom's house during late winter, when the weather was still unpredictable. We had sun but it was muddy from the snowmelt, so we had the ceremony in my mom's house. Erica was given my Grandma Annie's Indian name—Eshe-vat, "Walking Woman." Hence, Erica became a member of the Medicinebull family, and her new, adopted mother is a Cheyenne chief's daughter.

Erica's moves back to California and later to Iowa were difficult ones, but our family understood that while her time spent with us on a daily basis had ended, it would not be the end but meant that we would keep in contact via long distance—phone calls, e-mail, shorter visits, etc. Erica's last visit was last summer (2008); she and her husband showed our family their firstborn son, and my mother also gave her son a Cheyenne name. We get picture updates and are happy to hear the latest news of him, and that he still has his red hair.

My time with Erica was a learning experience, and for me, it has been a great experience to have a "cultural exchange" centered on learning each other's cultural background, more about this young white woman named Erica Prussing, and further about anthropology and her fieldwork at Northern Cheyenne.

Erica's fieldwork helped me to learn about anthropology, and particularly the focal point of her work, more so than the residents at Northern Cheyenne understand. I was impressed and pleased to read Erica's final manuscript for publication. Mainly, the older Cheyenne generation perspectives from the women were poignant and fascinating, as I am from the younger generation, but to read what the older women had experienced gives me profound inspiration and affirms my choice of an alcohol- and drug-free life.

There is controversy on the reservation regarding published works on the Cheyenne, and the general attitude about published works on the Cheyenne is abrasive. The typical Cheyennes believe that published works receive a huge sum of money, and that those Cheyennes who assist the authors receive a substantial amount of money as well. Another attitude is that written works by non-Indians about the Cheyenne promote unfavorable views of the people, which incites anger/resentment.

However, my personal view is that my Cheyenne grandparents accepted the white man's education, and they raised their children and strongly encouraged the grandchildren to attain an education. It was their view that education can help an individual to sustain a better way of living. Growing up with the encouragement of my grandparents and parents allowed me to have an open mind about education, and about the academics that come to the reservation and conduct their work with the Cheyenne. In addition, I have befriended a few academicians and agree with them on several areas, and, as a Cheyenne person, approve of them on a human level after studying them as they have come to the reservation to "study the Cheyenne." I trust my adopted sister Erica to be "human," and as an anthropologist/educator, she displays the compassion for Cheyenne people that is evident in her written work.

This reservation can be a difficult place to commit to a life of sobriety, but if an individual has the proper help/support from family/friends/community, it is a great place to live one's life and raise a family. I maintain my sobriety with the help of the sweat lodge, and the sweat lodge is my support system. The sweat lodge owners also believe that a spiritual foundation affirms an individual's commitment to a life of sobriety.

I learned and continue to learn to live my life in a balanced manner, and to be optimistic within my community, the Northern Cheyenne Reservation. There are "bad days" to go through and a wave of "good days" that give hope for a continued positive future. My group of support comes from Native spirituality and the sweat lodge, and the sweat lodge owners are committed to a life of sobriety and belief in a spiritual foundation of prayer and positive self-being.

Living each day to the best of our abilities with the resources and tools available here at Northern Cheyenne is challenging, as is a life of sobriety in any community. The difference here at Northern Cheyenne is that both sobriety and Native spirituality are possible, and an effective support system is available. I write this to convey a message to those individuals who choose to live a sober life while on the Northern Cheyenne Reservation. In the new stage after making this choice, they are vulnerable, because to maintain a sober life, they must let go of their drinking friends and are in need of friends who will support them in their decision of sobriety. If they do not make sober friends, then oftentimes they will eventually return to the alcohol/drug scene. My circle of friends or my new prayer family is who supports me in my sobriety, and my spirituality centers on the sweat lodge.

There have been several young people who attended the sweat and became regulars. Moreover, while participants may come and go, the sweat lodge maintains a consistently nonjudgmental and prayerful atmosphere. Those attending may be few at times, but when all show up on the same night, it will feel like no one was ever absent from the sweat.

I write this to those who may be new, to encourage you and to inform you that the first several months will be the toughest test of learning to live a sober lifestyle here on the rez; however, there are individuals/groups who live a sober lifestyle for many years. The key is to find the right group of individuals that will work for you. There are individuals who practice the 12 Steps of Alcoholics Anonymous, and this process works for them (and that is fine), and others combine Cheyenne spirituality with A.A. New individuals attend the sweat lodge, and we encourage them to practice and perhaps seek what is most beneficial for them. If what they are seeking is a place in the community where other individuals use Cheyenne spirituality of their own accord, then it is a good place to become a regular attendee.

Notes

CHAPTER 1

1. All research participant names are pseudonyms.

2. I have not been able to determine the date when it was founded, but a Native American Indian General Service Office of Alcoholics Anonymous has also been developed within Alcoholics Anonymous, with a website available at: http://www.naigso-aa.org/.

3. These studies pose a number of interesting questions. Borovoy (2005) suggests that an incipient political consciousness accompanies transformations in Japanese women's subjectivity as they consider the application of "codependency" to their interpersonal relationships. Brandes (2002) explores the ways in which Mexican men's A.A. meetings serve distinct social and cultural purposes, including both the maintenance and transformation of conventional Mexican masculinity. Similar inquiries into gender, power, and subjectivity are relevant for Native communities, but gender issues have rarely been emphasized in studies of Native North American sobriety, especially with regard to women (cf. Baird-Olson and Ward 2000), making these questions especially timely.

CHAPTER 2

1. Originally called Dull Knife Memorial College and now called Chief Dull Knife College, this tribal college was founded in Lame Deer in the 1970s as part of a nationwide push by Native American activists for greater local control of higher education. The curriculum originally emphasized high school completion and vocational training, and later added two-year associate's degrees as well as several distance-learning programs through which students can earn bachelor's degrees without leaving the reservation.

2. I encountered this fact when assisting a writing instructor at the tribal college who wanted his students to interview community elders about the Battle of the Little Bighorn for an assignment. I soon realized that this topic was not going to elicit very detailed or rich material and later found that anthropologist Margot

Liberty had observed that "no coherent tribal memory of the years between 1850 and 1880 remains today" (Stands in Timber and Liberty 1998:160f).

3. Piercing involved being tethered to a pole with thongs attached to skewers that pierced the flesh of the chest and/or the back, and walking around the pole for a specified time period (often several days) until the skewers broke loose.

4. These areas were initially known by corresponding band names (e.g., White River, Ree, Little Wolf, Black Lodges, Northern Scabbies, and Totimana), but these terms soon entered into competition with the English names that predominate today: Busby, Muddy/Ree, Lame Deer, Birney, and Ashland. Most of the latter are names of early Indian agents and white settlers in the region. Lame Deer, the administrative center of the reservation, was named for a Lakota chief who had been killed in a battle with soldiers from Fort Keogh just south of town in 1877. "Muddy" refers to Muddy Creek, an offshoot of the larger Rosebud Creek that flows down from the Yellowstone River.

5. A number of sociologists and economists include Northern Cheyenne in their analyses of how institution-building impacts economic development in the era of self-governance (e.g., Cornell and Kalt 1992) and the development of human capital (e.g., Ward and Snipp 1996).

6. Interestingly, Powell reports that Dull Knife split off from Little Wolf's group and did not want to listen to the guidance of the visionary woman, asserting, "We are men . . ." (1969:209–210). I have not heard this gender-based disagreement reported elsewhere.

7. To my knowledge, the first woman elected to serve on the Tribal Council was Bessie Standing Elk Harris, who held this position for some years starting shortly after the council was established in 1934. Female council members do not seem to have been elected again until the 1970s, however.

8. Many of the key actors involving in planning and implementing these events have some degree of experience with sobriety, and with the discussions of historical and multigenerational trauma that have been developed by and for Native North American communities (see chapter 1).

9. Straus (1976) records how *crazy* was used as a Cheyenne-English term to designate behavior that falls outside of cultural norms. She also notes how drunks are often said to act crazy, as I discuss further in chapter 3.

10. Sun Dances include participants (pledgers and instructors), their supporters, and a variety of spectators. The majority of community members involved are spectators, and I am referring to their decisions to attend here. Pledgers and their supporters make such extensive preparations that it is not feasible for them to attend more than one Sun Dance.

11. One-half Cheyenne "blood" was initially required for enrollment. In subsequent decades this limit was revised to one-quarter. In the 1960s enrollment criteria were redefined as descendance from a tribal member who appeared in

the 1935 enrollment census. In the 1990s blood quantum levels still appeared on tribal identity cards and were recorded in tribal enrollment databases, however.

12. Beginning in the 1960s, community leaders like John Woodenlegs sought funding to develop Cheyenne language and cultural curricula for use starting in elementary schools. By the 1970s a tribally run community college had been established in Lame Deer (Dull Knife Memorial College, later renamed Chief Dull Knife College). Richard Littlebear, a Northern Cheyenne tribal member who holds a doctorate, began serving as president of the college in the 1990s and spearheaded further language revitalization efforts. The founding of a locally controlled public high school on the reservation in 1995 has also offered new possibilities for such programs.

13. Some scholars translate *Tsitsistas* as "Sand People" or "Desert People" (e.g., Straus 1976:320), but there is considerable debate over the meaning and origin of the term (e.g., Moore 1999:146). There is general consensus among scholars that the *Chaiena* term originated in the Lakota language, from a term that means "Red Talkers," or people who speak a foreign tongue (Weist 1977:14). *Chaiena* seems to have become "Cheyenne" in the lingua franca of the Plains region in subsequent eras and, ultimately, in American English.

14. I use the masculine pronoun here since in all known nineteenth-century examples, exiled tribal members were male (Llewellyn and Hoebel 1941). Llewellyn and Hoebel elaborate that there were circumstances that mitigated the exile of the murderer, such as self-defense and, interestingly, drunkenness, but that the renewal ceremony was required in all cases of homicide (1941:166–168).

15. In some regards women do seem to have been subject to restraints upon emotional expression that parallel those applied to men. Grinnell records the ideal that one select a woman who is even-tempered to oversee the finishing touches of raising a lodge, lest the lodge always be smoky (1972a:229)!

16. Male pledgers and instructors were central to both Arrow Worship and Sun Dance, although the wife of the pledger enacted an important role as Sacred Woman during the latter. Less has been recorded about the Massaum ceremony, but Grinnell was present during the last performance of this ritual among the Northern Cheyennes in 1911 (1972b:285–336; see also Aadland 1996), and anthropologist Karl Schlesier (1987) reconstructed the ceremony based on work among the Southern Cheyennes. The main pledger for the Massaum was female (Moore 1999:230).

17. There are also specific terms for wine and beer in Cheyenne, which roughly translate to "that which tastes sweet" and "boiling/exploding water," respectively (see, for example, Northern Cheyenne Title VII Bilingual Education Program 1976).

CHAPTER 3

1. Such attentive biocultural studies have been conducted for some Native American health issues such as diabetes (e.g., Benyshek 2005), but not yet in significant numbers for alcohol use.

2. Soon after the town of Buffalo, Wyoming, was founded in 1879, for example, it was home to 637 people—and 17 saloons (Smith 1966:3).

3. Many early studies focused on the local cultural meanings and purposes served by the heavier binge-drinking styles that were cast as deviant in conventional popular perceptions and psychiatric standards (e.g., Kemnitzer 1972; Kunitz and Levy 1974; Topper 1980). Key studies such as Lurie (1971) also considered the political dimensions of these local systems of meaning, by suggesting that Native drinking could actually serve as one means of articulating Native identity in a world of major constraints imposed on such expression. While demonstrating that drinking serves important social and cultural functions could be read as an effort to minimize its adverse effects (Spicer 1997), most ethnographers have been careful to note the serious economic, social, and physical suffering that alcohol can produce in Native communities (Heath 1983; Kunitz and Levy 1994).

4. Some Northern Cheyennes do seem to believe that Native peoples have an innate predisposition to drink excessively, yet there also seems to be considerable controversy on this point (see also Kunitz and Levy 1974). Those pursuing sobriety, with whom I work most closely, tend to view drinking as more of a learned behavior or a habit, and as a result see laws as helpful adjuncts in encouraging people to become aware that their drinking leads to negative consequences.

5. For these details about the history of local alcohol services, special thanks are due to Charles Bearcomesout and Christine Valentine. Any mistakes are my own.

6. One man I know went through the detox program a full 50 times before eventually staying sober. These "revolving door" kinds of stories are certainly not unique to Northern Cheyenne but echo accounts from alcohol programs in both Native and non-Native communities (Kunitz and Levy 1994:196).

7. The possession and use of a stone (often red pipestone) pipe indicates that one has special rights and responsibilities in relation to spiritual powers. The smoke from such a pipe offers one's promises and pledges to the Creator. If one subsequently fails to fulfill these, then uncontrolled—and therefore dangerous (see Moore 1999:212)—spiritual energy is released.

PART II

1. Some affirm these insights by relating unresolved experiences of suffering to an absence of coherent narrative, noting the literal as well as figurative

unspeakability of some traumatic experiences, and suggesting that such representations are more accurately viewed as non-narrative "chaos" accounts (Frank 1995) or "chronicles" (Spicer 1998).

CHAPTER 4

1. Interestingly, the narratives of Northern Cheyenne men involved in Twelve Step recovery include more frequent references to feelings of shame generated by living on the margins of non-Native society, often in describing why and how they started drinking. John Bing of Emory University has conducted an ethnographic study emphasizing Northern Cheyenne men's experiences with alcohol, and use of local ritual practices in support of sobriety.

CHAPTER 5

1. The narrative of Belle Highwalking, recorded by Katherine (Toby) Weist in the 1970s, includes similar themes.

2. Northern Cheyenne tribal leaders and courts have implemented stronger policies for dealing with sex offenders during the past 10 years, although community members who work in schools and other contexts that involve mandatory reporting of child abuse continue to express frustration with how some chronic perpetrators seem to experience few or no legal consequences.

CHAPTER 7

1. Reports issued by IHS at the national level offer intriguingly different portraits of how tribal governance systems impact health care. Rhoades et al. noted the "excellent infrastructure" (1988:627) available for community-based prevention activities for alcoholism, and identified the key barrier to the success of such programs as community attitudes and support. More recent works that are aimed at a similar audience of practitioners and program planners, such as the selections in Nebelkopf and Phillips (2004), offer more complex portraits.

Works Cited

Aadland, Dan
  1996 Women and Warriors of the Plains: The Pioneer Photography of Julia
  E. Tuell. Missoula, MT: Mountain Press.
Abbott, Kathryn A.
  1999 Alcohol and the Anishinaabeg of Minnesota in the Early Twentieth
  Century. Western Historical Quarterly 30(1):25–43.
Abu-Lughod, Lila
  1986 Veiled Sentiments: Honor and Poetry in a Bedouin Society. Berkeley:
  University of California Press.
Adams, Alyce
  2000 The Road Not Taken: How Tribes Choose between Tribal and Indian
  Health Service Management of Health Care Resources. American Indian
  Culture and Research Journal 24(3):21–38.
Adelson, Naomi
  2000 Being Alive Well: Health and the Politics of Cree Well-being. Toronto:
  University of Toronto Press.
Alcoholics Anonymous
  2002 Alcoholics Anonymous: The Story of How Many Thousands of
  Men and Women Have Recovered from Alcoholism. 4th ed. New York:
  Alcoholics Anonymous World Services.
American Psychiatric Association
  1994 Diagnostic and Statistical Manual of Mental Disorders: DSM-IV. 4th
  ed. Washington, DC: American Psychiatric Press.
Anderson, Jeffrey D.
  2001 The Four Hills of Life: Northern Arapaho Knowledge and Life
  Movement. Lincoln: University of Nebraska Press.
Antze, Paul
  1987 Symbolic Action in Alcoholics Anonymous. *In* Constructive Drinking:
  Perspectives on Drink from Anthropology. Mary Douglas, ed. Pp. 149–181.
  New York: Cambridge University Press.

Armstrong, Elizabeth
  2003 Conceiving Risk, Bearing Responsibility: Fetal Alcohol Syndrome
  and the Diagnosis of Moral Disorder. Baltimore: Johns Hopkins University
  Press.
Asad, Talal, ed.
  1995 Anthropology and the Colonial Encounter. Amherst, NY: Prometheus
  Books.
Bacigalupo, Ana Mariella
  2007 Shamans of the Foye Tree: Gender, Power and Healing among
  Chilean Mapuche. Austin: University of Texas Press.
Baird-Olson, Karren, and Carol Ward
  2000 Recovery and Resistance: The Renewal of Traditional Spirituality
  among American Indian Women. American Indian Culture and Research
  Journal 24(4):1–35.
Barnes, Linda L.
  1998 The Psychologizing of Chinese Healing Practices in the United States.
  Culture, Medicine and Psychiatry 22(4):413–443.
Bateson, Gregory
  1972 Steps to an Ecology of Mind: Collected Essays in Anthropology,
  Psychiatry, Evolution, and Epistemology. San Francisco: Chandler.
Beals, J., A. Belcourt-Dittloff, S. Freedenthal, C. Kaufman, C. Mitchell, N.
Whitesell, K. Albright, F. Beauvais, G. Belcourt, B. Duran, C. Fleming, N.
Floersch, K. Foley, L. Jervis, BJ Kipp, P. Mail, S. Manson, P. Mohatt May G, B.
Morse, D. Novins, J. O'Connell, T. Parker, G. Quintero, P. Spicer, A. Stiffman, J.
Stone, J. Trimble, K. Venner, and K. Walters
  2009 Reflections on a Proposed Theory of Reservation-Dwelling American
  Indian Alcohol Use: Comment on Spillane and Smith (2007). Psychological
  Bulletin 135(2):339–343.
Becker, Gay
  1997 Disrupted Lives: How People Create Meaning in a Chaotic World.
  Berkeley: University of California Press.
Behar, Ruth
  2003 Translated Woman. 2nd ed. Boston: Beacon Press.
Benyshek, Daniel C.
  2005 Type 2 Diabetes and Fetal Origins: The Promise of Prevention
  Programs Focusing on Prenatal Health in High Prevalence Native American
  Communities. Human Organization 64(2):192–200.
Berkhofer, Robert F.
  1978 The White Man's Indian: Images of the American Indian from
  Columbus to the Present. New York: Vintage Books.

Bezdek, Marjorie, and Paul Spicer
    2006 Maintaining Abstinence in a Northern Plains Tribe. Medical
    Anthropology Quarterly 20(2):160–181.
Biehl, Joao, Byron Good, and Arthur Kleinman, eds.
    2007 Subjectivity: Ethnographic Investigations. Berkeley: University of
    California Press.
Bird, S. Elizabeth
    1996 Dressing in Feathers: The Construction of the Indian in American
    Popular Culture. Boulder, CO: Westview Press.
Black, Claudia
    2001[1982] It Will Never Happen to Me: Growing Up with Addiction as
    Youngsters, Adolescents, Adults. 2nd ed. Bainbridge, WA: Mac Publishing.
Borovoy, Amy
    2005 The Too-Good Wife: Alcohol, Codependency, and the Politics of
    Nurturance in Postwar Japan. Berkeley: University of California Press.
Bourdieu, Pierre
    1990 The Logic of Practice. Palo Alto: Stanford University Press.
Brady, Maggie
    1995 Culture in Treatment, Culture as Treatment: A Critical Appraisal of
    Developments in Addictions Programs for Indigenous North Americans
    and Australians. Social Science and Medicine 41(11):1487–1498.
Brandes, Stanley
    2002 Staying Sober in Mexico City. Austin: University of Texas Press.
Brenneis, Donald
    2000 Identifying Practice: Comments on "The Pragmatic Turn in
    Psychological Anthropology." Ethos 27(4):530–535.
Briggs, Charles L.
    1986 Learning How to Ask: A Sociolinquistic Appraisal of the Role of the
    Interview in Social Science Research. New York: Cambridge University Press.
Brodwin, Paul
    2003 Marginality and Subjectivity in the Haitian Diaspora. Anthropological
    Quarterly 76(3):383–410.
Cain, Carole
    1991 Personal Stories: Identity Acquisition and Self-Understanding in
    Alcoholics Anonymous. Ethos 19(2):210–253.
Calloway, Colin G.
    1997 New Worlds for All: Indians, Europeans, and the Remaking of Early
    America. Baltimore: Johns Hopkins University Press.
Campbell, Gregory R.
    1989 The Epidemiological Consequences of Forced Removal: The Northern
    Cheyenne in Indian Territory. Plains Anthropologist 34(124):85–97.

Champagne, Duane
    1989 American Indian Societies: Strategies and Conditions of Political and
    Cultural Survival. Cambridge, MA: Cultural Survival.
    2007 In Search of Theory and Method in American Indian Studies.
    American Indian Quarterly 31(3):353–372.
Churchill, Ward
    1992 Fantasies of the Master Race: Literature, Cinema and the Colonization
    of American Indians. Monroe, ME: Common Courage Press.
Clifford, James, and George E. Marcus
    1986 Writing Culture: The Poetics and Politics of Ethnography. Berkeley:
    University of California Press.
Cohn, Bernard S.
    1996 Colonialism and Its Forms of Knowledge: The British in India.
    Princeton, NJ: Princeton University Press.
Comaroff, Jean, and John L. Comaroff
    2003 Ethnography on an Awkward Scale: Postcolonial Anthropology and
    the Violence of Abstraction. Ethnography 4(2):291–324.
Comaroff, John L., and Jean Comaroff
    1987 The Madman and the Migrant: Work and Labor in the Historical
    Consciousness of a South African People. American Ethnologist 14:191–209.
    1992 Ethnography and the Historical Imagination. Boulder: Westview
    Press.
Cornell, Stephen E., and Joseph P. Kalt, eds.
    1992 What Can Tribes Do? Strategies and Institutions in American Indian
    Economic Development. Los Angeles: American Indian Studies Center,
    University of California Los Angeles.
Coyhis, Don, and William L. White
    2002 Alcohol Problems in Native America: Changing Paradigms and
    Clinical Practices. Alcoholism Treatment Quarterly 20(3):157–165.
Crapanzano, Vincent
    1980 Tuhami: Portrait of a Moroccan. Chicago: University of Chicago Press.
Csordas, Thomas J.
    1999 Ritual Healing and the Politics of Identity in Contemporary Navajo
    Society. American Ethnologist 26(1):3–23.
Csordas, Thomas J., and Arthur Kleinman
    1996 The Therapeutic Process. In Medical Anthropology: A Handbook of
    Theory and Method. Carolyn F. Sargent and Thomas M. Johnson, eds.
    Pp. 11–25. New York: Greenwood Press.
Cultural Survival
    2007 Recognizing Indigenous Peoples' Human Rights, http://www.cultural
    survival.org (accessed Jan. 20, 2009).

Davies, Wade
    2001 Healing Ways: Navajo Health Care in the Twentieth Century.
    Albuquerque: University of New Mexico Press.
Deloria, Philip Joseph
    1998 Playing Indian. New Haven: Yale University Press.
Deloria, Vine
    1988[1969] Custer Died for Your Sins: An Indian Manifesto. Norman:
    University of Oklahoma Press.
Denzin, Norman K.
    1987 The Alcoholic Self. Beverly Hills: Sage.
Department of Health and Human Services
    2001 Surgeon General's Report, Mental Health: Culture, Race and Ethnicity
    (Supplement) (3/15).
Desjarlais, Robert, and Theresa D. O'Nell
    2000 Introduction: The Pragmatic Turn in Psychological Anthropology.
    Ethos 27(4):407–414.
Dippie, Brian
    1982 The Vanishing American: White Attitudes and U.S. Indian Policy.
    Lawrence: University of Kansas Press.
Dole, Christopher, and Thomas J. Csordas
    2003 Trials of Navajo Youth: Identity, Healing and the Struggle for
    Maturity. Ethos 31(3):357–384.
Dorris, Michael
    1990 The Broken Cord. New York: HarperPerennial.
Douglas, Mary, ed.
    1987 Constructive Drinking: Perspectives on Drink from Anthropology.
    New York: Cambridge University Press.
Duran, Eduardo E., and Bonnie Duran
    1995 Native American Postcolonial Psychology. Albany: State University of
    New York Press.
Durie, Mason
    1998 Whaiora-Māori Health Development. 2nd ed. London: Oxford
    University Press.
Eber, Christina
    2000 Women and Alcohol in a Highland Maya Town: Water of Hope,
    Water of Sorrow. Austin: University of Texas Press.
Edmunds, R. David
    1995 Native Americans, New Voices: American Indian History, 1895–1995.
    American Historical Review 100(3):717–740.
Fabian, Johannes
    1991 Time and the Work of Anthropology. London: Routledge.

Fadiman, Anne
     1997 The Spirit Catches You and You Fall Down: A Hmong Child, Her
     American Doctors, and the Collision of Two Cultures. New York: Farrar,
     Straus and Giroux.
Farmer, Paul
     1999 Infections and Inequalities: The Modern Plagues. Berkeley: University
     of California Press.
Fast, Phyllis Ann
     2002 Northern Athabascan Survival: Women, Community, and the Future.
     Lincoln: University of Nebraska Press.
Fingarette, Herbert
     1989 Heavy Drinking: The Myth of Alcoholism as a Disease. Berkeley:
     University of California Press.
Fixico, Donald L., ed.
     1997 Rethinking American Indian History. Albuquerque: University of
     New Mexico Press.
Frank, Arthur W.
     1995 The Wounded Storyteller: Body, Illness and Ethics. Chicago:
     University of Chicago Press.
Frank, John W., Roland S. Moore, and Genevieve M. Ames
     2000 Historical and Cultural Roots of Drinking Problems among
     American Indians. American Journal of Public Health 90(3):344–351.
Garro, Linda C., and Gretchen Chesley Lang
     1994 Explanations of Diabetes: Anishinaabeg and Dakota Deliberate
     upon a New Illness. In Diabetes as a Disease of Civilization: The Impact of
     Culture Change on Indigenous Peoples. Jennie R. Joe and Robert S. Young,
     eds. Pp. 293–328. New York: Walter de Gruyter.
Garroutte, Eva Marie
     2003 Real Indians: Identity and the Survival of Native America. Berkeley:
     University of California Press.
Gone, Joseph P.
     2006 Mental Health, Wellness, and the Quest for an Authentic American
     Indian Identity. In Mental Health Care for Urban Indians: Clinical Insights
     from Native Practitioners. Tawa M. Witko, ed. Pp. 55–80. Washington, DC:
     American Psychological Association.
     2008 The Pisimweyapiy Counselling Centre: Paving the Red Road to
     Wellness in Northern Manitoba. In Aboriginal Healing in Canada: Studies
     in Therapeutic Meaning and Practice. James Waldram, ed. Pp. 133–203.
     Ottawa: Aboriginal Healing Foundation.
     2009 A Community-Based Treatment for Native American Historical
     Trauma: Prospects for Evidence-Based Practice. Journal of Consulting and
     Clinical Psychology 77(4):751–762.

Good, Byron, and Mary-Jo DelVecchio Good
    1994 In the Subjunctive Mode: Epilepsy Narratives in Turkey. Social
    Science and Medicine 38(6):835–842.
    2003 Introduction: Culture in the Politics of Mental Health Research.
    Culture, Medicine and Psychiatry 27(4):369–71.
Good, Byron J., Mary-Jo DelVecchio Good, Sandra T. Hyde, and Sarah Pinto
    2008 Postcolonial Disorders: Reflections on Subjectivity in the
    Contemporary World. *In* Postcolonial Disorders. Mary-Jo DelVecchio
    Good, Sandra T. Hyde, and Sarah Pinto, eds. Pp. 1–40. Berkeley: University
    of California Press.
Good, Mary-Jo DelVecchio, Sandra T. Hyde, and Sarah Pinto, eds.
    2008 Postcolonial Disorders. Berkeley: University of California Press.
Goodman, Alan H., Deborah Heath, and M. Susan Lindee, eds.
    2003 Genetic Nature/Culture: Anthropology and Science beyond the Two-
    Culture Divide. Berkeley: University of California Press.
Grinnell, George Bird
    1956[1915] The Fighting Cheyennes. Norman: University of Oklahoma
    Press.
    1972a[1923]   The Cheyenne Indians, vol. 1: History and Society. Lincoln:
    University of Nebraska Press.
    1972b[1923]   The Cheyenne Indians, vol. 2: War, Ceremonies, and Religion.
    Lincoln: University of Nebraska Press.
Grossman, Roberta, dir.
    2005 Homeland: Four Portraits of Native Action. 90 min. Bullfrog Films.
    Oley, PA.
Guha, Ranajit, and Gayatri Spivak, eds.
    1988 Selected Subaltern Studies. New York: Oxford University Press.
Gusfield, Joseph R.
    1986 Symbolic Crusade: Status Politics and the American Temperance
    Movement. Urbana: University of Illinois Press.
Hahn, Robert A.
    1999 Anthropology and the Enhancement of Public Health Practice.
    In Anthropology in Public Health: Bridging Differences in Culture and
    Society. Robert A. Hahn, ed. Pp. 3–24. New York: Oxford University Press.
Hall, Roberta L.
    1986 Alcohol Treatment in American Indian Populations: An Indigenous
    Treatment Modality Compared with Traditional Approaches. Annals of the
    New York Academy of Sciences 474:168–178.
Hazelden
    2010 What Happens in Addiction Treatment? http://www.hazelden.org/
    web/public/whathappenstxt.page (accessed May 18, 2010).

Heath, Dwight B.

   1983 Alcohol Use among North American Indians: A Cross-Cultural Survey of Patterns and Problems. *In* Research Advances in Alcohol and Drug Problems. Reginald G. Smart, Frederick B. Glaser, Yedy Israel, Harold Kalant, Robert E. Popham, and Wolfgang Schmidt, eds. Pp. 7:343–396. New York: Plenum Press.

   2000 Drinking Occasions: Comparative Perspectives on Alcohol and Culture. Philadelphia: Brunner/Mazel.

Herman, Judith L.

   1992 Trauma and Recovery. New York: Basic Books.

Herzfeld, Michael

   1997 Cultural Intimacy: Social Poetics in the Nation-State. New York: Routledge.

   2001 Anthropology: Theoretical Practice in Culture and Society. Malden, MA: Wiley-Blackwell.

Hobsbawm, Eric, and Terence Ranger, eds.

   1983 The Invention of Tradition. New York: Cambridge University Press.

Hoebel, E. Adamson

   1978 The Cheyennes: Indians of the Great Plains. 2nd ed. New York: Holt, Rinehart and Winston.

Holland, Dorothy, and Kevin Leander

   2004 Ethnographic Studies of Positioning and Subjectivity: An Introduction. Ethos 32(2):127–139.

Holmes, Arthur, and George McPeek

   1988 The Grieving Indian. Minneapolis: Indian Life Ministries.

Hunt, Linda

   2000 Strategic Suffering: Illness Narratives as Social Empowerment among Mexican Cancer Patients. *In* Narrative and the Cultural Construction of Illness and Healing. Cheryl Mattingly and Linda C. Garro, eds. Pp. 88–107. Berkeley: University of California Press.

Inhorn, Marcia C.

   1994 Quest for Conception: Gender, Infertility and Egyptian Medical Traditions. Philadelphia: University of Pennsylvania Press.

Irvine, Leslie

   1999 Codependent Forevermore: The Invention of Self in a Twelve Step Group. Chicago: University of Chicago Press.

Jilek-Aall, Louise

   1981 Acculturation, Alcoholism and Indian-Style Alcoholics Anonymous. Journal of Studies on Alcohol 9(suppl.):143–158.

Johnson, Miranda

   2008 Making History Public: Indigenous Claims to Settler States. Public Culture 20(1):97.

Jones, David S.
  2003 Virgin Soils Revisited. William and Mary Quarterly 60:703–742.
  2004 Rationalizing Epidemics: Meanings and Uses of American Indian
  Mortality since 1600. Cambridge: Harvard University Press.
  2006 The Persistence of American Indian Health Disparities. American
  Journal of Public Health 96(12):2122–2134.
Kaminer, Wendy
  1992 I'm Dysfunctional, You're Dysfunctional: The Recovery Movement
  and Other Self-Help Fashions. New York: Perseus Books.
Kasl, Charlotte Davis
  1992 Many Roads, One Journey: Moving beyond the Twelve Steps. New
  York: HarperPerennial.
Kelm, Mary Ellen
  2004 Wilp Wa'Ums: Colonial Encounter, Decolonization and Medical Care
  among the Nisga'a. Social Science and Medicine 59(2):335–349.
Kemnitzer, Luis S.
  1972 The Structure of Country Drinking Parties on Pine Ridge Reservation,
  South Dakota. Plains Anthropologist 17:134.
Kessler, Donna J.
  1996 The Making of Sacagawea: A Euro-American Legend. Tuscaloosa:
  University of Alabama Press.
Kilpatrick, Jacquelyn
  1999 Celluloid Indians: Native Americans and Film. Lincoln: University of
  Nebraska Press.
Kirmayer, Laurence J.
  2000 Broken Narratives: Clinical Encounters and the Poetics of Illness
  Experience. *In* Narrative and the Cultural Construction of Illness and
  Healing. Cheryl Mattingly and Linda C. Garro, eds. Pp. 153–180. Berkeley:
  University of California Press.
Kirmayer, Laurence J., Gregory M. Brass, and Caroline L. Tait
  2000 The Mental Health of Aboriginal Peoples: Transformations of Identity
  and Community. Canadian Journal of Psychiatry 45(7):607–616.
Kleinman, Arthur
  1988 The Illness Narratives: Suffering, Healing and the Human Condition.
  New York: Basic Books.
Kleinman, Arthur, and Peter Benson
  2006 Anthropology in the Clinic: The Problem of Cultural Competency
  and How to Fix It. PLoS Medicine 3(10):1673–1676.
Kleinman, Arthur, Veena Das, and Margaret Lock, eds.
  1997 Social Suffering. Berkeley: University of California Press.

Kleinman, Arthur, and Joan Kleinman
  1997 The Appeal of Experience, the Dismay of Images. *In* Social Suffering. Arthur Kleinman, Veena Das, and Margaret Lock, eds. Pp. 1–24. Berkeley: University of California Press.
Kohrt, Brandon A., and Ian Harper
  2008 Navigating Diagnoses: Understanding Mind–Body Relations, Mental Health, and Stigma in Nepal. Culture, Medicine and Psychiatry 32(4):462–491.
Krauss, Deborah
  1991 Regulating Women's Bodies: The Adverse Effects of Fetal Rights Theory on Childbirth Decisions and Women of Color. Harvard Civil Rights–Civil Liberties Law Review 26(2):523–548.
Kunitz, Stephen J.
  2000 Globalization, States and the Health of Indigenous Peoples. American Journal of Public Health 90(10):1531–1539.
Kunitz, Stephen J., and Jerrold E. Levy
  1974 Changing Ideas of Alcohol Use among Navajo Indians. Quarterly Journal of Studies on Alcohol 35:243–259.
  1994 Drinking Careers: A Twenty-Five-Year Study of Three Navajo Populations. New Haven: Yale University Press.
Langness, Lewis L., and Gelya Frank
  1981 Lives: An Anthropological Approach to Biography. Novato, CA: Chandler and Sharp.
Lavoie, Josée G.
  2004 Governed by Contracts: The Development of Indigenous Primary Health Services in Canada, Australia and New Zealand. Journal of Aboriginal Health 1(1):6–24.
Lee, Sing, and Arthur Kleinman
  2007 Are Somatoform Disorders Changing with Time? The Case of Neurasthenia in China. Psychosomatic Medicine 69(9):846–849.
Leland, Joy
  1976 Firewater Myths: North American Indian Drinking and Alcohol Addiction. New Brunswick: Publication Division, Rutgers Center of Alcohol Studies.
Levy, Jerrold E., and Stephen J. Kunitz
  1974 Indian Drinking: Navajo Practices and Anglo-American Theories. New York: John Wiley and Sons.
Lewin, Ellen, and William L. Leap, eds.
  1996 Out in the Field: Reflections of Lesbian and Gay Anthropologists. Urbana: University of Illinois Press.

Lindenbaum, Shirley, and Margaret Lock, eds.
  1993 Knowledge, Power, and Practice: The Anthropology of Medicine and Everyday Life. Berkeley: University of California Press.
Lindholm, Charles
  2007 Culture and Identity: The History, Theory and Practice of Psychological Anthropology. Oxford: Oneworld.
Linger, Daniel T.
  1994 Has Culture Theory Lost Its Minds? Ethos 22(3):284–315.
Llewellyn, Karl N., and E. Adamson Hoebel
  1941 The Cheyenne Way: Conflict and Case Law in Primitive Jurisprudence. Norman: University of Oklahoma Press.
Lock, Margaret, and Patricia Kaufert, eds.
  1998 Pragmatic Women and Body Politics. New York: Cambridge University Press.
Lock, Margaret, and Nancy Scheper-Hughes
  1996 A Critical-Interpretive Approach in Medical Anthropology: Rituals and Routines of Discipline and Dissent. In Handbook of Medical Anthropology. Carolyn F. Sargent and Thomas M. Johnson, eds. Pp. 41–70. Westport, CT: Greenwood Press.
Lucas, Phil, dir.
  1985 The Honour of All. 56 min. Filmwest Associates. Canada.
Lurie, Nancy O.
  1971 The World's Oldest On-Going Protest Demonstration: North American Indian Drinking Patterns. Pacific Historical Review 40:311–332.
MacAndrew, Craig, and Robert B. Edgerton
  1969 Drunken Comportment: A Social Explanation. Chicago: Aldine.
Mader, Jerry
  2002 The Road to Lame Deer. Lincoln: University of Nebraska Press.
Madsen, William
  1974 The American Alcoholic: The Nature–Nurture Controversy in Alcoholic Research and Therapy. Springfield, IL: Charles C. Thomas.
  1979 Alcoholics Anonymous as a Crisis Cult. In Beliefs, Behaviors and Alcoholic Beverages. Mac Marshall, ed. Pp. 382–387. Ann Arbor: University of Michigan Press.
Mail, Patricia D., and David R. McDonald
  1980 Tulapai to Tokay: A Bibliography of Alcohol Use and Abuse among Native Americans of North America. New Haven: HRAF Press.
Makela, Klaus, ed.
  1996 Alcoholics Anonymous as a Mutual-Help Movement: A Study in Eight Societies. Madison: University of Wisconsin Press.

Mancall, Peter C.
    1995 Deadly Medicine: Indians and Alcohol in Early America. Ithaca:
    Cornell University Press.
Manson, Spero M.
    1997 Ethnographic Methods, Cultural Context, and Mental Illness:
    Bridging Different Ways of Knowing and Experience. Ethos 25(2):249–258.
Marcus, George E., and Michael M. J. Fischer, eds.
    1986 Anthropology as Cultural Critique: An Experimental Moment in the
    Human Sciences. Berkeley: University of California Press.
Marquis, Thomas B.
    1978 The Cheyennes of Montana. Algonac, MI: Reference Publications.
Marquis, Thomas B., Margot Liberty, and John Woodenlegs
    2007 A Northern Cheyenne Album. Norman: University of Oklahoma
    Press.
Marshall, Mac, ed.
    1979 Beliefs, Behaviors and Alcoholic Beverages: A Cross-Cultural Survey.
    Ann Arbor: University of Michigan Press.
Marshall, Mac, and Leslie Marshall
    1990 Silent Voices Speak: Women and Prohibition in Truk. Belmont, CA:
    Wadsworth.
Marshall, Mac, and Alice Oleson
    1996 MADDer than Hell. Qualitative Health Research 6(1):6–22.
Mattingly, Cheryl
    1998 Healing Narratives and Clinical Plots: The Narrative Structure of
    Experience. Cambridge: Cambridge University Press.
Mattingly, Cheryl, and Linda C. Garro, eds.
    2000 Narrative and the Cultural Construction of Illness and Healing.
    Berkeley: University of California Press.
May, Philip A.
    1982 Substance Abuse and American Indians: Prevalence and Susceptibility.
    International Journal of the Addictions 17(7):1185–1209.
    1994 The Epidemiology of Alcohol Abuse among American Indians: The
    Mythical and Real Properties. American Indian Culture and Research
    Journal 18(2):121–143.
McDonald, Maryon, ed.
    1994 Gender, Drink and Drugs. Providence, RI: Berg.
Medicine, Bea
    2007 Drinking and Sobriety among the Lakota Sioux. Lanham, MD: Alta
    Mira Press.

Mezzich, Juan E., Laurence J. Kirmayer, Arthur Kleinman, Horatio Fabrega Jr.,
Delores L. Parron, Byron J. Good, Keh-Ming Lin, and Spero M. Manson
    1999 The Place of Culture in DSM-IV. Journal of Nervous and Mental
    Disease 187(8):457–464.
Mihesuah, Devon A., and Angela C. Wilson, eds.
    2004 Indigenizing the Academy: Transforming Scholarship and
    Empowering Communities. Lincoln: University of Nebraska Press.
Miller, John Clark
    2008 12-Step Treatment for Alcohol and Substance Abuse Revisited: Best
    Available Evidence Suggests Lack of Effectiveness or Harm. International
    Journal of Mental Health and Addiction 6:568–576.
Moore, John H.
    1987 The Cheyenne Nation: A Social and Demographic History. Lincoln:
    University of Nebraska Press.
    1999 The Cheyenne. Cambridge, MA: Blackwell.
National Association for Native American Children of Alcoholics
(NANACOA)
    2005 White Bison, NANACOA, http://www.whitebison.org/nanacoa/his
    tory.html (accessed Jan. 31, 2005).
Nebelkopf, Ethan, and Mary Phillips, eds.
    2004 Healing and Mental Health for Native Americans: Speaking in Red.
    Walnut Creek, CA: AltaMira Press.
Nichter, Mark, and Margaret Lock, eds.
    2002 New Horizons in Medical Anthropology: Essays in Honour of
    Charles Leslie. London: Routledge.
Noren, Jay, David Kindig, and Audrey Sprenger
    1998 Challenges to Native American Health Care. Public Health Reports
    113(1):22–33.
Northern Cheyenne Title VII Bilingual Education Program
    1976 English–Cheyenne Student Dictionary. Lame Deer: Northern
    Cheyenne Language and Culture Center.
Oaks, Laury
    2001 Smoking and Pregnancy: The Politics of Fetal Protection. New
    Brunswick: Rutgers University Press.
Ohnuki-Tierney, Emiko, ed.
    1990 Culture through Time: Anthropological Approaches. Stanford:
    Stanford University Press.
O'Nell, Theresa D.
    1996 Disciplined Hearts: History, Identity and Depression in an American
    Indian Community. Berkeley: University of California Press.

2000   "Coming Home" among Northern Plains Vietnam Veterans: Psychological Transformations in Pragmatic Perspective. Ethos 27(4):441–465.

2004   Culture and Pathology: Flathead Loneliness Revisited. Culture, Medicine and Psychiatry 28:221–230.

O'Nell, Theresa D., and Christine M. Mitchell

1996   Alcohol Use among American Indian Adolescents: The Role of Culture in Pathological Drinking. Social Science and Medicine 42(4):565–578.

Ortner, Sherry

2006   Anthropology and Social Theory: Culture, Power and the Acting Subject. Durham, NC: Duke University Press.

Paradies, Yin C., Michael J. Montoya, and Stephanie M. Fullerton

2007   Racialized Genetics and the Study of Complex Diseases: The Thrifty Genotype Revisited. Perspectives in Biology and Medicine 50(2):203–227.

Parish, Steven M.

2008   Subjectivity and Suffering in American Culture: Possible Selves. New York: Palgrave Macmillan.

Pearce, Roy Harvey

1988[1962]   Savagism and Civilization: A Study of the Indian and the American Mind. Berkeley: University of California Press.

Peele, Stanton

1989   Diseasing of America: Addiction Treatment Out of Control. Lexington, MA: Lexington Books.

1993   The Conflict between Public Health Goals and the Temperance Mentality. American Journal of Public Health 83(6):805–810.

Penny, H. Glenn

2006   Elusive Authenticity: The Quest for the Authentic Indian in German Public Culture. Comparative Studies in Society and History 48(4):798–818.

Personal Narratives Group

1989   Interpreting Women's Lives: Feminist Theory and Personal Narratives. Bloomington: Indiana University Press.

Peters, Stella A.

1992   Hi! Cheyennes: My Nursing Years at Lame Deer, Montana. Bozeman, MT: Color World Printers.

Powell, Peter J.

1969   Sweet Medicine: The Continuing Role of the Sacred Arrows, the Sun Dance, and the Sacred Buffalo Hat in Northern Cheyenne History. Norman: University of Oklahoma Press.

1981   People of the Sacred Mountain: A History of the Northern Cheyenne Chiefs and Warrior Societies, 1830–1879: With an Epilogue, 1969–1974. New York: Harper and Row.

Prussing, Erica
    2007 Reconfiguring the Empty Center: Drinking, Sobriety and Identity in
    Native American Women's Narratives. Culture, Medicine and Psychiatry
    31(4):499–526.
    2008 Sobriety and Its Cultural Politics: An Ethnographer's Perspective
    on "Culturally Appropriate" Addiction Services in Native North America.
    Ethos 36(3): 354–375.
Quintero, Gilbert
    2000 "The Lizard in the Green Bottle": "Aging Out" of Problem Drinking
    among Navajo Men. Social Science and Medicine 51:1031–1045.
    2001 Making the Indian: Colonial Knowledge, Alcohol and Native
    Americans. American Indian Culture and Research Journal 25(4):57–71.
Quintero, Gilbert, and Mark Nichter
    1996 The Semantics of Addiction. Journal of Psychoactive Drugs
    28:219–228.
Rapp, Rayna
    1999 Testing Women, Testing the Fetus: The Social Impact of
    Amniocentesis in America. New York: Routledge.
Rhoades, Everett R., Russell D. Mason, Phyllis Eddy, Eva M. Smith, and
Thomas R. Burns
    1988 The Indian Health Service Approach to Alcoholism among American
    Indians and Alaska Natives. Public Health Reports 103(6):621 627.
Rodin, Miriam B.
    1985 Getting on the Program: A Biocultural Analysis of Alcoholics
    Anonymous. In The American Experience with Alcohol: Contrasting
    Cultural Perspectives. Linda A. Bennett and Genevieve M. Ames, eds. Pp.
    41–58. New York: Plenum Press.
Ross, Fiona C.
    2001 Speech and Silence: Women's Testimonies in the First Five Weeks
    of Public Hearings of the South African Truth and Reconciliation
    Commission. In Remaking a World: Violence, Social Suffering, and
    Recovery. Veena Das, Arthur M. Kleinman, Margaret Lock, Mamphela
    Aletta Ramphele, and Pamela Reynolds, eds. Pp. 250–280. Berkeley:
    University of California Press.
Sadler, Patricia O.
    1979 The "Crisis Cult" as a Voluntary Association: An Interactional
    Approach to Alcoholics Anonymous. In Beliefs, Behaviors and Alcoholic
    Beverages: A Cross-Cultural Survey. Mac Marshall, ed. Pp. 388–393. Ann
    Arbor: University of Michigan Press.
Said, Edward
    1978 Orientalism. New York: Vintage Books.

Scheper-Hughes, Nancy

  1992 Hungry Bodies, Medicine, and the State: Toward a Critical
  Psychological Anthropology. *In* New Directions in Psychological
  Anthropology. Theodore Schwartz, Geoffrey M. White, and Catherine A.
  Lutz, eds. Pp. 221–247. New York: Cambridge University Press.

Schlesier, Karl H.

  1987 The Wolves of Heaven: Cheyenne Shamanism, Ceremonies, and
  Prehistoric Origins. Norman: University of Oklahoma Press.

Schwarz, Maureen Trudelle

  1995 The Explanatory and Predictive Power of History: Coping with the
  "Mystery Illness," 1993. Ethnohistory 42(3):375–401.

Shoemaker, Nancy, ed.

  2002 Clearing a Path: Theorizing the Past in Native American Studies.
  London: Routledge.

Simonds, Wendy

  1992 Women and Self-Help Culture: Reading between the Lines. New
  Brunswick: Rutgers University Press.

Singer, Merrill

  2008 Drugging the Poor: Legal and Illegal Drugs and Social Inequality.
  Long Grove, IL: Waveland Press.

Singer, Merrill, and Hans Baer

  1995 Critical Medical Anthropology. Amityville, NY: Baywood.

Smith, Andrea

  2005 Conquest: Sexual Violence and American Indian Genocide.
  Cambridge, MA: South End Press.

Smith, Helena Huntington

  1966 The War on Powder River. New York: McGraw-Hill.

Smith-Morris, Carolyn

  2005 Diagnostic Controversy: Gestational Diabetes and the Meaning of
  Risk for Pima Indian Women. Medical Anthropology 24(2):145–177.

Sobo, Elisa J.

  2009 Culture and Meaning in Health Services Research: A Practical Field
  Guide. Walnut Creek, CA: Left Coast Press.

Spicer, Paul

  1997 Toward a (Dys)Functional Anthropology of Drinking: Ambivalence
  and the American Indian Experience with Alcohol. Medical Anthropology
  Quarterly 11(3):306–323.

  1998 Narrativity and the Representation of Experience in American
  Indian Discourses about Drinking. Culture, Medicine and Psychiatry
  22(2):139–169.

  2001 Culture and the Restoration of Self among Former American Indian
  Drinkers. Social Science and Medicine 53:227–240.

Stands in Timber, John, and Margot Liberty
1998 Cheyenne Memories. 2nd ed. New Haven: Yale University Press.
Stepan, Nancy
1982 The Idea of Race in Science: Great Britain, 1800–1960. London: Macmillan.
Storm, Hyemeyohsts
1972 Seven Arrows. New York: Harper and Row.
Straus, Anne S.
1976 Being Human in the Cheyenne Way. Ph.D. dissertation, University of Chicago.
1977 Northern Cheyenne Ethnopsychology. Ethos 5(3):326–357.
Substance Abuse and Mental Health Administration
2005 Gathering of Native Americans (GONA) Curriculum, http://p2001 .Health.org/CTI05/Ctio5ttl.Htm (accessed January 31, 2005).
Swora, Maria Gabrielle
2001 Commemoration and the Healing of Memories in Alcoholics Anonymous. Ethos 29(1):58–77.
Taylor, Janelle
2003 The Story Catches You and You Fall Down: Tragedy, Ethnography, and "Cultural Competence." Medical Anthropology Quarterly 17(4):159–181.
Topper, Martin D.
1980 Drinking as an Expression of Status: Navajo Male Adolescents. In Drinking Behavior among Southwestern Indians: An Anthropological Perspective. Jack O. Waddell and Michael W. Everett, eds. Pp. 103–147. Tucson: University of Arizona Press.
U.S. Department of the Interior, National Park Service
2009 Sand Creek Massacre National Historic Site, http://www.nps.gov/ sand/index.htm (accessed January 15, 2009).
Van Hollen, Cecilia
2003 Birth on the Threshold: Childbirth and Modernity in South India. Berkeley: University of California Press.
Waldram, James B.
1997 The Way of the Pipe: Aboriginal Spirituality and Symbolic Healing in Canadian Prisons. Peterborough, Ontario: Broadview Press.
2004 Revenge of the Windigo: The Construction of the Mind and Mental Health of North American Aboriginal Peoples. Toronto: University of Toronto Press.
Walle, Alf H.
2004 The Path of Handsome Lake: A Model of Recovery for Native People. Charlotte, NC: Information Age Publishing.

Ward, Carol J.
    2005 Native Americans in the School System: Family, Community, and
    Academic Achievement. Lanham, MD: Alta Mira Press.
Ward, Carol J., Gregory Hinckley, and Kae Sawyer
    1995 The Intersection of Ethnic and Gender Identities: Northern Cheyenne
    Women's Roles in Cultural Recovery. In American Families: Issues in Race
    and Ethnicity. Cardell K. Jacobson, ed. Pp. 201–227. New York: Garland.
Ward, Carol J., and C. Matthew Snipp, eds.
    1996 Human Capital and American Indian Economic Development.
    Greenwich, CT: JAI.
Ward, Carol J., and David R. Wilson
    1989 Educational Census of the Northern Cheyenne Reservation. n.p.
Warry, Wayne
    1998 Unfinished Dreams: Community Healing and the Reality of
    Aboriginal Self-Government. Toronto: University of Toronto Press.
Weibel-Orlando, Joan
    1989 Hooked on Healing: Anthropologists, Alcohol, and Intervention.
    Human Organization 48(2):148–155.
    1999[1991] Indian Country, L.A.: Maintaining Ethnic Community in
    Complex Society. Urbana: University of Illinois Press.
Weist, Katherine
    1971 The Northern Cheyennes: Diversity in a Loosely Structured Society.
    Ph.D. dissertation, University of California at Berkeley.
    1982 Belle Highwalking: The Narrative of a Northern Cheyenne Woman.
    Billings: Montana Council for Indian Education.
Weist, Thomas D.
    1977 A History of the Cheyenne People. Billings: Montana Council for
    Indian Education.
    1978 Editor's introduction. In The Cheyennes of Montana. Thomas B.
    Marquis. Pp. 9–22. Algonac, MI: Reference Publications.
White, William L.
    1998 Slaying the Dragon: The History of Addiction Treatment and
    Recovery in America. Normal, IL: Chestnut Health Systems.
Wilcox, Danny M.
    1998 Alcoholic Thinking: Language, Culture, and Belief in Alcoholics
    Anonymous. Westport, CT: Praeger.
Wilkins, David E., and K. Tsianina Lomawaima
    2002 Uneven Ground: American Indian Sovereignty and Federal Law.
    Norman: University of Oklahoma Press.
Zarowsky, Christina
    2004 Writing Trauma: Emotion, Ethnography, and the Politics of Suffering
    among Somali Returnees in Ethiopia. Culture, Medicine and Psychiatry
    28:189–209.

Index

abandonment, 69, 129, 130, 131, 181

abstinence, 87, 92, 106, 144–145, 191

accreditation, 88, 210, 211–212

addiction research and treatment, 2, 15, 16, 19, 87, 88, 171, 182

Adult Children of Alcoholics (ACOA): on alcoholic families, 183; emergence of, 15–16; psychological transformation emphasized by, 178; Recovery Center services influenced by, 90; terms and concepts from, 98, 109, 129, 131; Twelve Step approaches and, 86

Al Anon, 15, 82

alcohol, Cheyenne terms for, 10, 31, 66, 243n17

alcoholic (term), label questioned, 92, 190; recovering, 15; self-identification as, 12, 68, 94

"alcoholic families" (concept), 129, 144, 182–183

Alcoholics Anonymous (A.A.): alcoholism (concept), 5, 12, 15, 85, 92; Anglo orientation of, 16; anthropological studies of, 18; Cheyenne women's involvement in, 18, 82, 123, 178, 188; emergence of, 12; history of Cheyenne participation in, 82

alcohol-related problems: biological explanations for, 73–75; deaths from, 23, 129, 150; defining and addressing, 27, 90, 93, 230; illnesses, 22, 75; limitations and pitfalls of diagnostic labels, 91; perceived Native predisposition for, 73, 79, 244n4; psychosocial explanations for, 74, 75, 80; women's perceptions of, 105–106

alcohol-related violence: historic accounts of, 77; local histories of, 23; older women's accounts of, 122–123, 150; women's concerns over, 85; younger women's accounts of, 129, 131–133, 143

alcohol services: challenges of, 227; cultural barriers to, 224–226; culturally appropriate, 4, 7–10, 19, 28, 70, 201–203, 232; diversity and, 3–4, 85, 200; emergence on reservation, 78–79, 81–82

alcohol use: Cheyenne attitudes concerning, 9, 19, 35, 71, 76, 83, 94; colonization and, 3, 17, 20, 31; diversity of Native, 73, 75; forms of, 91; history of, 72, 74–75, 76–82; impact of, 21–22; laws concerning, 9, 74–75, 79–80; moral erosion and, 119–125, 163; motives for, 136–137; Native American stereotypes and, 10, 11, 73, 75; normal *versus* pathological, 4, 8, 78, 81, 84, 85; prevalence and impact of, 133–134; rise in, 1–2, 78–82, 94, 98, 120, 143;

address, 31, 200, 205; perception as problem, 67; personal and collective well-being impacted by, 1–2; recognizing, 227
social authority: Cheyenne language and, 60; debates about, 3, 49, 56, 59, 92–93, 102; and link to cultural identity, 36–37, 49; politics of, 107
social inequalities: in anthropology, 23–24; as colonial legacy, 5; "Indian drinking" and, 72–73; "Indian" image role in, 61; non-Native unawareness of, 29; reproduction of, 201; rhetorical frameworks for, 222
spiritual practices, Cheyenne. *See* ritual/spiritual practices, Cheyenne
Stands in Timber, John, 38, 53, 65, 77–78
Straus, Anne (Terry), 33
subjectivity, 100, 101, 104–107, 231
substance abuse: ethnographic research on, 227–228; services for, 7, 201, 202, 229
substance use: kinship ties impacted by, 164–165; normative, 82–90; overview of, 84; as recreation, 135; by younger women, 134
Sun Dances: Cheyenne language use in, 60; controversies concerning, 56; criminalization of, 59; women's involvement in, 189, 193, 195, 197, 198
sweat lodges, 193, 197, 198, 231, 239, 240
Sweet Medicine (culture hero), 39, 46, 52, 198
Sweet Medicine prophecies and teachings: on alcohol, 78, 147; on Cheyenne identity, 37, 55, 57; current problems interpreted through, 50; of early reservation

life, 51; fatalistic *versus* inspirational interpretations of, 53, 54; on peaceable conduct, 63; on sacred objects, 50; on trajectory of loss, 61

Tallbull, Bill, 38, 53
Timber, Stephanie (pseudonym), 234–236
tradition (concept): culture and, 222–223; generational differences in perceptions of, 125; local meanings and debates surrounding, 6, 55, 57; older women's attitudes concerning, 114
tribal enrollment, 58–59, 137–138
Tribal Health Services: and dealings with Indian Health Service, 88, 207, 217–218, 220–221, 235, 236; federal funding through, 203, 206; as local control agency, 86; self-determination and, 208–221, 230
Twelve Step approaches and therapies: advocates of, 7, 10, 27, 97, 99, 143–144, 184, 199, 240 (*see also* younger women, Twelve Step involvement of); alternatives to, 87, 93, 188; anthropological studies of, 18; Cheyenne cultural heritage and, 189–190, 194; content of, 13; criticism concerning, 7, 14, 27, 29, 70–71, 91; cultural conflicts with, 17, 18, 184–185, 200, 225–226; discourse and practice, 12–18; effectiveness of, 6; emphasis on abstinence, 92; modifications of, 4, 5, 6–7, 18, 19, 90, 95, 97, 173, 174, 179, 190–191, 193, 195, 228; Protestant traditions and, 16; reliance on, 17–18, 78, 81, 82, 87–88; sexual abuse discussions and, 123. *See also* Recovery Center, Twelve Step approaches at

About the Author

Erica Prussing is Assistant Professor of Anthropology and Community and Behavioral Health at the University of Iowa. She earned a Ph.D. in anthropology from the University of California at San Diego, and an M.P.H. specializing in epidemiology from the University of California at Berkeley. She completed postdoctoral training in mental health services and health outcomes research at Children's Hospital and Health Center in San Diego. Her recent publications about sobriety on the Northern Cheyenne Reservation appear in *Ethos* and *Culture, Medicine and Psychiatry*. Her current research examines how anthropology can shed critical light on the concepts and reasoning used in epidemiology, and provides an international comparison of how indigenous peoples are increasingly using community-based epidemiological research to achieve greater local control in defining and addressing their health needs.